MW01657079

Praise for *Because I Remember Terror, Father, I Remember You*

"[Silverman's] lyric style transforms a ravaged childhood into a work of art. . . . The book reads like a poem."—*St. Petersburg Times*

"This harrowing memoir gives voice to the inarticulate terror Silverman suffered as a child, when she could never find the right words to describe her situation. She has found them now."—*Booklist*

"Searing, brave, powerfully written. . . . Sue Silverman's memoir is about more than incest: it is about evil, about denial, about the great chasm between the public facade of a prominent, successful family and its painful reality, and it is about how, as in a Greek tragedy, a curse has been passed down through several generations. This book is the cry that shatters the curse."—ADAM HOCHSCHILD

"Riveting. Scalding. Brilliant."—SYD LEA

"Beautiful, rocketing prose."—*Tallahassee Democrat*

"A disturbing story . . . told in a way designed to sear itself into your soul."—*Lansing State Journal*

"If you doubt, read this book. If you're stuck, read this book. If you're numb, read this book. For it will pound into you that incest is real, that it is awful and that it happens everywhere, in every corner of society, behind some of the prettiest front doors."—*Healing Woman*

"[Sue William Silverman's] writing is almost too beautiful in describing the horrors. . . . She writes in an eloquent but bare-bones style."—*Sojourner: The Women's Forum*

"Heartwrenching . . . beautifully crafted."—*Austin American-Statesman*

"The evocative detail makes it all the more disconcerting."—*Cleveland Plain Dealer*

"A difficult subject in the hands of a skilled writer."—*Lansing Capital Times*

"Harrowing and heartbreaking."—*Grand Rapids Press*

"Extraordinary . . . vivid . . . written in perfect clarity. . . . I applaud Silverman for her remarkable psychological journey back to a chance at a healthy future."—*Kliatt*

"Searing . . . riveting . . . compelling."—*Omaha World-Herald*

"So vivid that it stirred more than a few of my own demons. . . . [Silverman's] words scream the truth and her journey is real and powerful."—*Full Circle News*

"A harrowing memoir of incest and survival."—*Feminism, Philosophy, and the Law*

Also by Sue William Silverman

Love Sick: One Woman's Journey through Sexual Addiction

Because I Remember Terror, Father, I Remember You

Winner of the Associated Writing Programs Award

for Creative Nonfiction

Because I Remember Terror, Father, I Remember You

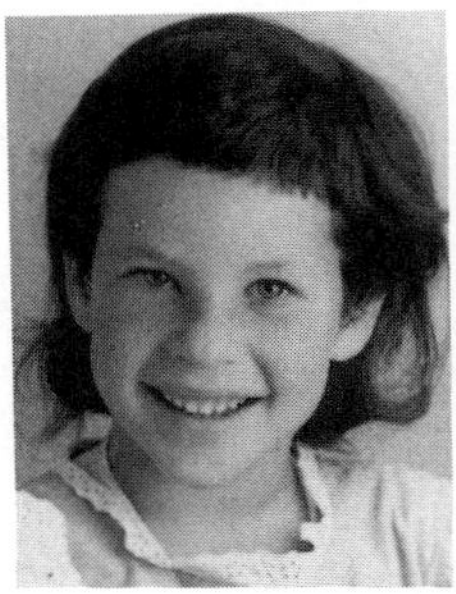

SUE WILLIAM SILVERMAN

The University of Georgia Press
Athens and London

University of Georgia Press paperback edition, 1999
Published by the University of Georgia Press
Athens, Georgia 30602

Designed by Sandra Strother Hudson
Set in Fournier by Books International, Inc.
Printed and bound by Maple-Vail
The paper in this book meets the guidelines for permanence
and durability of the Committee on Production Guidelines
for Book Longevity of the Council on Library Resources.

Printed in the United States of America

06 07 08 09 10 P 11 10 9 8 7

The Library of Congress has cataloged
the hardcover edition of this book as follows:
Library of Congress Cataloging-in-Publication Data
Silverman, Sue William.
Because I remember terror, Father, I remember you /
Sue William Silverman.
xv, 272 p. ; 22 cm.
ISBN 0-8203-1870-1 (alk. paper)
1. Silverman, Sue William. 2. Adult child sexual abuse victims—
United States—Biography. 3. Adult child abuse victims—
United States—Biography. I. Title.
HV6570.2 .S55 1996
362.7'64'092—dc20 96-13706
[B]

Paperback ISBN-13: 978-0-8203-2175-2
ISBN-10: 0-8203-2175-3

British Library Cataloging-in-Publication Data available

www.ugapress.org

For Mack, with My Love
and
To Randy, for My Life

The limits of my language mean the limits of my world.

WITTGENSTEIN

Contents

Acknowledgments

I am deeply grateful to:

Adam Hochschild, and D.W. Fenza and the Associated Writing Programs, for selecting my book for the 1995 creative nonfiction award;

Malcolm Call, for his insight, generosity, and courage;

Charles East, for his honesty and wisdom;

Michele Orwin, Naomi H. Wittes, and Nancy Lord, who faithfully accompanied my book on its journey.

Preface

From 1933 to 1953 my father was Chief Counsel to the Secretary of the Interior. He was architect of the preliminary papers establishing statehood for Alaska and Hawaii. He assisted in the plans for Philippine independence, helped create the Puerto Rican Commonwealth, and worked to implement home rule for the Virgin Islands, Guam, and Samoa. He also helped establish civilian rule of Japanese possessions after World War II. From 1954 to 1958 my father was president of the West Indies Bank and Trust Company. After leaving the West Indies, he became president of the Saddle Brook Bank and Trust Company in New Jersey. I have photographs of my father with President Harry Truman, Adlai Stevenson, Governor Richard J. Hughes of New Jersey, Senator Henry "Scoop" Jackson.

My father was also a child molester. I know. Because he sexually molested me.

Prologue: I Remember You, Father

How can I help you?" Randy Groskind asks.

This is the first question Randy, a therapist in Atlanta, asks me when I enter his office. I'm too tired to answer. I sit rigid on a couch and stare at the plant by the window, wishing I were small enough, light enough, to curl up inside one of the cool green leaves and sleep. This exhaustion—I feel the actual dense weight of the answer to his question. My head feels too heavy to think. My mouth feels too heavy to speak.

I wonder: Do I extract the first snapshot from my mind in order to be lighter? Extract the first image, all the images that flip through my mind like snapshots. Not photographs. One lingers over photographs, studying shadows and patterns of light. The tongue slows over the three long syllables of "photograph" with time to study faces, relationships, with time to understand what the picture means. But a snapshot is a glance. Quickly, the tongue slaps the roof of the mouth, whispering "snap," whispering "shot." Then the snapshot implodes in my mind—a secret no one, I've told myself, should see. Over the years I've glimpsed fragments of these snapshots, but in the past months they are relentless. So it is now, finally, I want to capture the image: hold it, hold it, hold it. This is why I'm here in Randy's office. For now, I believe, I must see a photograph of what my father did to me, see what he did to my body. And because I see terror, Father, I see and I remember you.

I see this. It is 1962. New Jersey. My boyfriend has just finished a wrestling match, and I sit in his red Rambler, crammed between high school friends, smelling the sweaty gym on our clothes. It's a late-winter afternoon, already dark. Outside the car window the school yard is frozen, white with snow. My family has moved here from the West Indies, and at first I missed Caribbean colors. But now I'm comforted by blankness, by ice, by white. Comforted by thick winter clothes cloaking my body, by the furry lining of my suede jacket, soft under my chin. Steam fogs the windows. This comforts me, too, for if I stay in this car forever no one will see me; no one will be able to touch me. But as the car turns a corner toward my home my friends' bodies press against me. Suddenly I no longer hear their voices. I no longer hear sound. This pressure. This smell of sweat. I am no longer in this car. I think I will stop breathing.

I am in my bedroom of baby-blue walls with matching spread and ruffle. The room is decorated with faded gardenia corsages from school dances, paper Hawaiian leis, silver ribbons and glass beads, red satin hearts with gold glitter—a young teenager's room. But in the deepest moment of night, the room grays. No, wait. On my headboard is a six-inch plastic Christmas tree—a toy. Every night my father winds it. Red, green, blue, white lights sweep the ceiling and walls, closer, the bed, as the tree revolves, closer, revolves flecks of light on my body. The tree will unwind, finish, stop, before he does. Globes of light darken. The snapshot blackens to negative. *You're right, Father. No one will ever see us. No one will ever know.*

I glance at Randy. Is he the one who will finally see me, who will finally know? Is he the one to whom I can entrust the snapshots of my secret mind? But if Randy sees them, if he sees me, surely he'll think I'm terrible, evil, unworthy. He won't want me to return to his office again, ever.

How can I help you? he'd asked me.

Randy is quiet. His office is quiet. The soft gaze of his blue eyes soothes me. I wonder which snapshots I must reveal in order for him to understand the exhaustion.

Patiently he awaits an answer.

RED

The Egyptian Princess

Washington, D.C.: 1950

I am four and pretend I am an Egyptian princess. For this game I arrange planks of wood across my parents' brown-and-white checked bedspread. The wood becomes a tributary of the Nile River, and as I flee along the bank, escaping, green reeds brush my legs. Someone is chasing me. Downstairs in the living room my father builds furniture with his electric saw, a gleaming metal table with a round, jagged blade, whirring as it nears the wood, whirring as it severs a plank gripped in a vise. I believe I hear the wood screaming, the metal slicing faster. I run faster. Metal slits my back. The blade against bare skin. My father accidentally cuts his hand on the blade and there is blood everywhere. I must slip off the bank to wash in the river because I see it: blood on my body. The Egyptian princess is gone.

□ □ □

I fold and refold my handkerchiefs. I trace a finger across white embroidered initials on lace: *SWS*. I press my face against a handkerchief decorated with pink flowers as if I can smell them. A blue and red handkerchief shows cartoon pictures of "Blondie." I have a magenta handkerchief with a white filigree design. I love all my pretty handkerchiefs. But because I can't bear to soil them, I never use them. Yet I still hand-wash each one in the sink. I watch them dry. When my mother sets up her ironing board I stand on a stool and iron and re-iron each handkerchief until it's perfect. I'm scared I might iron wrinkles *into* the material, rather than iron wrinkles out. As I iron I sprinkle the cotton with water stored in one of my father's old bay rum aftershave bottles that my mother saved for her ironing water. The residue of bay rum scent makes me dizzy. I don't understand why the scent reminds me of nightmares, reminds me of night. Of metal blades. Of an Egyptian princess fleeing. I try to concentrate on ironing my handkerchiefs. This is all. It is an imperative that the handkerchiefs be perfect.

I spend hours organizing my bureau until it is neat and perfect, too. I arrange ribbons, anklets, undershirts, scraps of lace from my mother's sewing kit. I have seven pairs of underpants with the names of days embroidered in different colors: red for Monday, yellow for Tuesday, green for Wednesday, pink for Thursday . . . White for Sunday. This pair scares me. Sundays scare me. I bury it under the pile of underwear. Maybe if I lose this pair . . . maybe if I never wear Sunday again. . . .

Except when he travels, my father is home all day Sunday. We go for outings in our black Chevrolet. While my mother learns to drive, my father is in a rage because she drives too slowly, wavering along country roads in Virginia. The car is hot and stifling. The gray felt seat feels scratchy under my thighs. My sister Kiki, two and a half years older than I, fidgets. She rolls the window up, down. She snaps the lid of the ashtray on the rear armrest. She will not speak to me. She will not smile at me. Usually Kiki disappears for hours to avoid me, avoid all of us. So today, trapped with her family, she must pretend she is far away from us all.

In the trunk is a wicker basket with a picnic lunch. Later, when we stop to eat, my father will fault sandwiches too warm, chicken not cooked right, deviled eggs not creamy enough. My father turns his wrath first on the food, then on the ants, then on the heat, then on us. The woman and two girls will sit in silence on a pretty checkered blanket, scared to object. No—my mother and I will sit in silence. My sister will wander off to a nearby stream. Or she will climb a tree—one precariously high—with no fear for her safety, while I am scared of everything, especially scared something bad will happen to my sister. And while I long to be like her, I know I never will be. Or, I wish I could bask in the reflected glory of my brave sister's ability to climb the highest tree or sneak out the back door into the alley after dark. But I am ignored by her, and the more I persist, the more insistently I am refused.

My mother makes a stab at fun on our Sunday outing. She teaches my sister and me a song: "Whistle while you work. / Hitler is a jerk. / Mussolini is a meany . . ." We sing rounds: "Row, row, row your boat . . ." My father does not join in. My sister's voice will be the first to fade, then my mother's. Finally, my thin voice trails to a slow halt. I sigh and close my eyes. Or stare up at the roof of the car. If I look down I'll get carsick and throw up. Please, don't let me throw up. I hate to eat; I hate to brush my teeth; I hate to throw up. I don't understand why my mouth hates to feel anything inside it—sometimes not even words. I can be speechless for hours, and if I concentrate hard enough I can pretend I don't have a mouth.

But on this particular Sunday we don't reach a picnic site. Even if my father is silent, his rage is not. He's not in control of the car and he has to be, he must be. My mother must feel this rage, radiating like heat against glass. Perhaps the steering wheel scorches her fingers. Perhaps a white searing light blinds her eyes. Slowly we drift onto the shoulder. Beneath the tires I sense soft, tentative ground. The car wobbles. Then it topples down an embankment, rolling over and over. I hear glass shatter and feel the sun strike my face. I pitch against my sister, sharp elbows and knees. Green smells of the gouged earth tumble past the crash of metal.

When the car is still I see treetops and sky. I am breathing. We all are breathing, collapsed against smashed windows and dented doors. My parents ask if we, their two daughters, are all right. Yes, we say, fine really. They don't think to check for major injury. But perhaps they wouldn't know where or how to actually inspect for damage anyway. A moment later, comforting hands reach for me—a woman's hands—helping me from the car window. It is these hands that gently examine my body for bruises or broken bones. But the touch is not scary; it is concerned and caring.

Our house is silent. In our family we don't know words to soothe each other's hurts; we lack a vocabulary designated for comfort. My mother is in the bedroom with the door shut. I know she is under the covers, the curtains drawn, her eyes closed and sleeping. My sister slips out the back door to play in the alley. And I—I trudge up the stairs to my bedroom and lie on my bed, trying to imagine the Egyptian princess. But today I'm too exhausted to imagine fleeing along the banks of the Nile. Today, my dolls and my handkerchiefs don't interest me. I hear my father follow up the wood stairs, this the only sound in the house. His steps are slow and measured. I imagine his hand skimming the rail. He probably plans to check on my mother, but he passes the door to her room. I wonder if she hears him, hears his footsteps pass her room and near mine.

My door is open. I lie on my side, and I glance at him as he stands in the doorway. I am surprised to see him. It is still early, way too early for him to kiss me good-night. His lips are parted—at first I think he's smiling—so I smile back, but his lips are too tight to smile. Until I do. Then his soften. And my smile—mine—I believe this is why he now enters my room. My smile is an invitation for him, *for you, Daddy. I'm happy to see you.* He must know this. *I* believe this, believe he continues to walk toward me because I smile.

He sits on the bed and strokes my back, this now the only sound, the friction of his hand on cotton. But for a moment so quick it is barely time, I feel—no, rather, it is my *body* that realizes—the difference between the way the woman had touched me earlier and his touch now. His touch—*his*—feels more like a stranger's touch than hers, the stranger's, had. There is a distance, a coolness to his touch, and I wish it were the woman still stroking me. He curls up beside me, his stomach against my back, and holds me tight-tight against him. His breath disturbs the hair at the nape of my neck. "I love you," he whispers. I believe he does this because I have smiled, he does this because he loves me. Yes, he loves me so much. He holds me tighter. His breath is harder. His tongue—I feel the tip of his tongue on my neck. His fingers grip my chin, and I think of the vise on his electric saw that grips the wood, steadily turning my face toward his. His tongue feels scary inside my . . . but I have forgotten the word for that part of my face. Moments later I imagine my mouth itself has disappeared. I'm not awake, I am sleeping, and I am tumbling down an embankment, not to the ground, but through time and space. I am the Egyptian princess. Exhausted, no longer able to flee, I have fallen asleep believing I am hidden in a deep thicket of reeds by the bank of the Nile River.

But wait. I am wrong. I *am* taught a definition for the word "comfort." I learn this from my father, learn this and many other things from him. I learn that I am able to comfort my father, console him when he is hurt, when he is sick.

And I learn I will never hear my mother's voice calling to me—Sue, Sue—my name as soft as a dove murmuring—Sue—the three small letters that mean me. But surely my name is too faint for me to hear my mother calling, wanting to save me—and I, the Egyptian princess, am too far away—as she whispers to me from the other side of the bedroom wall.

Or maybe I don't hear my mother because my name is no longer Sue. I am no longer Sue. Maybe I can't hear her because I have a new name now, a treasured name, for a girl who's a ruby, for a girl who's a pearl. A girl my father surely believes is more beautiful than ordinary, everyday Sue. *This* must be why I never hear my mother call: Sue, Sue, Sue.

□ □ □

When I am four, my mother begins to examine my Monday, Tuesday, Wednesday, Thursday underpants. She opens my bureau and removes each pair, inspects them, then sticks them back in the drawer, not neatly folded as before. Once, she pulls down the Monday underpants I am wearing and touches the crotch of the pants as they lie bunched around my ankles. I don't know why she does this. I'm afraid she'll find what she's looking for. And even though I don't know what this is, I know it is bad.

□ □ □

When I am older I study photographs in the family album. A Jamaican woman, Mrs. Robinson, a nurse or nanny, dressed in white, holds me. I am still an infant. She is smiling—proud of me? It would not be like our family to hire a nanny. My mother doesn't work. We don't have much money. Why do we need this woman? When I first begin to speak, I have a Jamaican accent. Where is my mother? Is she asleep in bed even now, years before the car crash?

In another photograph I stand across the street from our house, holding the rail of a metal fence, the boundary of a cemetery. My eyes are closed as the wind blows my short curls about my face. I want to ask that child why her eyes are closed. But I can't ask her: I don't dare to know what she knows, see what she's seen. Other photographs show young sisters in pinafores with white socks and black patent-leather shoes. Two sisters sit on the grass with their mother, picking clover to weave into a chain.

There is one small photograph in the family album I stare at again and again. It is of me, from the waist up, black and white, but dark, with little contrast. A veil of light filters my face. I wear a white sweater. I lie on my back, my arms crossed up over my shoulders, cradling my head. It looks awkward, posed—a slightly adult pose. I am expressionless, staring straight into the lens, but I'm not sure if it's *my* expression, or *my* face.

For there is another little girl. She has my face, but not my face; she has my body, but not my body. She is Dina. *She* is the girl my father most loves. She is the one to stare into the lens of the camera held by my father as he leans closer and closer to her body.

□ □ □

An excerpt from my father's journal kept while he was Chief Counsel to the Interior Department. Entry dated August 5, 1947. Occasion, the signing, by President Truman, of the Philippine independence papers:

> Called Congressman Crawford and arranged to meet him at White House at noon. Matt Connelly and Charley Ross showed us in precisely at 12:15. We circled the President seated ready to sign the bill. Dozens of cameramen were around taking pictures of the signing. The president seemed disturbed. It was shortly after his mother's death. He signed the bill with 4 different pens. He dated the Bill "Approved—July 5th." We called it to his attention. He said: "I don't know what's happening to me these days." We chatted a bit about the measure. We shook hands and left to have lunch with Oscar at Interior. Sat next to Crawford at lunch. He has a great interest in Puerto Rico. I am of the opinion he will do everything in his power to help the economy of the Island.

□ □ □

An excerpt from a letter dated December 15, 1949, to my mother from my father. He is on a government trip to the Pacific islands and Japan, where he stays in the Imperial Hotel in Tokyo:

> Another very curious sight is seeing so many of the Japanese wearing masks—the kind used for colds. They wear these masks out in the streets, to prevent the spreading of colds. Everything here is calculated in terms of spreading disease. They are terribly conscious of it. They do not shake hands. Those that do have gotten into the Stateside habit. They take their shoes off when they come into the house so as not to bring the street dirt into the house. We're told they rarely kiss—even parents and children rub cheeks or noses, but no kissing. I don't know what they would think of Suzie's tongue kissing. It's strictly non-Japanese.

Heartbeats in Stone

Bethesda, Maryland: 1951–1953

In Washington, D.C., we lived in a two-family house on Southern Avenue. Now, when I am five, we move into a ranch house on Kingswood Road in the suburbs. How proud my parents are of their brand-new home, the first they've ever purchased. How beautiful are the hardwood floors with Oriental rugs from Israel. My father tells me what a lucky little girl I am, with my own private bedroom, the windows high, close to the ceiling, so no one can see inside. The secluded living room overlooks a dark forest. Now my father has a shed, detached from the house, for his electric saw. How lucky he is to be able to saw undisturbed for hours.

My father brings us trinkets from business trips. Presents from Occupied Japan gleam like red lacquer. Philippine presents seem as green as the crown of a palm. Hawaiian presents are sweet-smelling leis and rustly grass skirts. Alaska is glittery snow and ice. Siam sparkles like silver and gold bangly jewelry. The Pacific Trust Territories and the West Indies smell like the azure and sapphire sea. I treasure fragile dolls from Bangkok, pink and black papier-mâché masks from Hong Kong, Eskimo totem poles, puppets, silk scarves scented with incense. I even save the wrapping paper, pressing it to my face and breathing deeply, imagining myself far away, although knowing I could never travel.

I would be afraid to travel. Instead I lie in bed, safe in my high-windowed bedroom, daydreaming of foreign countries, of what's outside, while my sister is the one to disappear into the world, escaping our house. I can't leave the house, for it might disappear while I'm gone. I imagine bricks crumbling, the roof and eaves lifted by gusts of wind to tumble to the farthest corner of sky. Beams will splinter and crack. Windows shatter. This is my fear. Only the unrelenting strength of my watchful gaze can prevent this disaster.

When my father returns home he is pleased to see me, the daughter who always waits for him, the daughter who knows how to make him happy. On Saturday he builds a dollhouse from construction paper. I cut out paper dolls to live inside. In the afternoon my mother cooks chicken and rice, fresh vegetables, an apple pie. The house smells right. But even though the day has been perfect, we grow silent around the dinner table. We—we three little girls, as my father always calls us, *his* three little girls—watch, without eating, watch while my father tests the food. The chicken must be crisp and dry, almost burned, or my father won't eat it. I breathe slowly before he takes his first bite, waiting to see the outcome of the meal. If he doesn't like the food, his rage will spew across the table to my mother and he will slam from the house to the shed, to his electric saw, sawing his rage through planks of plywood or pine.

Tonight, for my father, the food is fine. I eat little of the dry chicken but as much apple pie as possible. My sister, too, eats little, while my mother comments on whether she thinks we're eating the right amount, informing us of the nutritional value of each item of food and why our bodies need it. My mother worries so much about my body, always concerned it be sufficiently nourished. Vitamins. Minerals. Roughage. These are all it needs, surely she believes, in order to be healthy.

□ □ □

Always, I wait for my sister to invite me to play. I wait for her to come home, wait for her to speak to me, wait for her to notice me, smile at me, love me. But there doesn't seem to be enough of her to share herself with me. Her thin stick of a body barely stirs the air in the house. She has nothing to spare. I don't remember the sound of her voice; she is absent, even when here. Once, when her friend visits, I hide under the bed in her room to be close to her, as if I am part of them. Changing position, I bump my head. She screams at me, and I rush from the room in shame.

□ □ □

My report card from kindergarten, handwritten in pen by my teacher, indicates that I play alone much of the time and that when other students, usually boys, want a toy I'm playing with I relinquish it immediately. The teacher thinks I'm too passive. Yet during the year I show two signs of rebellion. Once I am discovered in a corner hammering a toy mallet against the ground. I refuse to stop when asked. The teacher calls this a "useless motion." Later in the year I am asked to open my mouth for a throat inspection by a visiting doctor. I refuse.

By second grade I no longer refuse requests concerning my body. For a school photograph I hold a crayon in my left hand and smile into the camera. I wear my most beautiful lime-green dress with white ruffles on the shoulder cuffs. My teacher takes the crayon from my left hand and puts it in my right. I tell her I'm left-handed, but she refuses for the photo to be taken unless the crayon is in my right hand. I comply.

□ □ □

I begin elementary school at the Alta Vista School in Montgomery County, Maryland. The long corridors, the endless doors and rooms, are large and scary. The cloakroom is moist with melting snow and mud. I sit on the floor in the corner to pull off my leggings. Other children laugh and push and shout, fighting over hooks upon which to hang parkas. Galoshes are kicked against the wall. The cloakroom darkens in this claustrophobic crush of children. In the small, warm room all the children seem to be melting. This crush, this dampness, is familiar, but I don't remember where else I feel it or smell it. But I am also my own opposite: After the other children leave the cloakroom, I *like* being here by myself. Then I sit on the floor against the wall, hidden behind coats and scarves. No one can see me. Now the darkness is comforting. Since I believe that what my mother searches for on my underpants is a smell that means I've been bad, I believe here no one can smell me. So I sit here until I am told to come out.

Always, I'm scared to come out. I'm scared to speak in school, scared to be noticed. All day I drink only small amounts of water, since I'm scared to ask for permission to use the bathroom. I'm scared to answer questions, even if I know the answers. Exhausted by fear, I'm unable to concentrate and fail to understand instructions on painting, on playing, on learning lessons. I feel almost foreign, as if I speak a different language. Always, I make mistakes. When reprimanded by a teacher I stare at my shoes, believing if I can't see her, then soon, in just one moment, she will no longer see me either. All through elementary school, teachers say I'm afraid to try new things. I know about new things. But it would never occur to me to tell anyone about the new things I am taught by my father.

□ □ □

The summer between first and second grade I am to attend daycamp. My fear of leaving my house deepens into fear of leaving my mother, deepens into numbing panic. I believe she is the only one on earth able to protect me—protect me from the image of the scared Egyptian princess. But I have no words for this image. I don't understand why the princess hides, so I can't explain what the image means. All I know is that if I don't watch my mother she, along with my house, will disappear. Now I imagine feet and ankles sinking below ground. Hair will snag in beaks of low-flying birds. Severed arms and hands will drift to the farthest horizon of space. My unrelenting gaze is all that holds my mother onto the skin of the earth. And if I lose her, the Egyptian princess will be . . . I don't know the word for what will happen.

On the first day of camp my mother pushes me into the car. Driving there I beg her not to make me go and think of excuses why she must need me at home. I'll help her cook and clean and iron. I'll wash every dish after dinner. I plead, but she doesn't understand the fear and I lack the appropriate vocabulary to explain it. When we arrive, the counselor and my mother both tug me from the car. Edged around the door is ropy trim, and I dig my fingers into it, holding on, kicking, screaming, crying. Boys watch while they pretend to play touch football, but my desperation not to stay outweighs any fear of being noticed. Finally I am pried loose, and my mother quickly drives away.

Now I am quiet. I am exhausted, bereft, stubborn. Not even the death of my mother would make me feel more abandoned. I sit on the ground and watch the boys play football. The counselor asks if I want to join girls beading necklaces. I shake my head, no, looking down, afraid to see him, afraid for him to see me, wanting, yes, to be invisible. Do I want to go horseback riding? Again I shake my head. Swimming? All I want—doesn't he know?—all I want to do is scream. I can't, I can't understand why he doesn't know what's wrong, why he can't fix this, even though I don't know what "this" is either. I am enraged he doesn't see what's invisible, enraged he can't hear words I'm unable to speak, enraged he can't smell the fear that evaporates on my skin by morning, every morning before I leave the house.

I watch the boys throw the football, watch as one boy catches it, watch the others tackle him. Surely the boy is crushed, his bones splintered, under the mound of kicking boys. Even when the boys peel themselves away and the boy who'd caught the ball stands, grinning, I'm not convinced he hasn't been hurt. I'm still not convinced, even as he breaks from the crowd, running. His hand rises high above his head, drifting back behind his shoulder before whipping forward, releasing the ball. It begins to arc, and without conscious will or plan I am off the ground and racing toward it. The ball soars across a green horizon, across the cool blue basin of sky. I run faster. Now *I* am the one to catch the ball. I grip the leather, holding on. The strong, noisy boys must hurry. They must. I will not relinquish it until I am on the very bottom of that crushing knot of boys.

Finally they tackle me, as I knew they would. This is what I want. Instead of feeling the weight of boys piled on top of me, I am weightless, free, far lighter than my body. Now it is my body able to twine with sunbeams high across the sky. No longer will my body have to be here, be trapped here. For I hear something crack—or maybe I feel it, although the feeling is far from pain. The crack in my collarbone is soothing, as if the marrow of bone seeps from its skeletal structure, warming me, healing me. Now my mother must pick me up from the camp. Now I need never go back.

□ □ □

I watch *The Mickey Mouse Club* on television and want to be Annette Funicello. To myself, I pretend my name is Annette and also name all five of my dolls Annette. But when I meet a girl named Anita I want her name, too. I have an urgent need for these names, to *be* these names, and spend days transforming myself into Annette or Anita, whispering these names to myself, chanting them like a mantra, trying to shed my own self, my own image.

Around the corner lives my best friend. We watch animals at the National Zoo. We play in a sandbox and roller-skate around the neighborhood. But I'm not close to her, not really. No real person enters my consciousness. I collect names of people, not people themselves. I steal their names, wanting truly to be their names more than I want to be them, for I'm not sure I want to be anybody.

□ □ □

I am in the bathtub, in this house on Kingswood Road. For hours, it seems, I stare at my yellow rubber duck with a blue sailor cap on its head. It bobs as my father moves his arm through the water. He holds a bar of white soap. He asks me to raise an arm. He washes my underarm, my neck, my chest. I smile up at him, the soapy water warm and slick across my skin. He moves the soap down my chest and across my stomach. He tickles my belly button and I giggle, before he moves the soap down farther, farther. It is between my legs. Gently, he edges my legs apart. The soap slips from his hand, and it is the soap I watch now, bobbing to the surface. He touches me there with a finger, in a place I can't name. In a place I have no name for, for no word exists. I will never let myself know the word, except it is a place, simply "down there." My giggle stops. His breath is so heavy it seems to ripple the water into the thinnest of waves. His fingers massage it. And it feels good, yes. I discover pleasure before I discover its shame, discover that the definition for pleasure is the definition of the word "shame."

□ □ □

In second grade I stop attending school. I refuse. No one understands why, so the school arranges for a psychologist to see me. This cheerful woman sits in a schoolroom, gives me four plastic dolls, and asks me to explain who they are. Here, I say, is a daddy doll in a business suit who loves his daughters very much. Here, I say, holding up a doll with a bright pink blouse, is a mommy doll, who also loves her daughters. And here is a beautiful sister doll who loves her younger sister. The youngest doll is a happy doll, I say, smiling: See her here in her pretty yellow dress. We are a happy family, I say, with absolute conviction, knowing with certainty that happiness implies I will never be taken away from my family. Yet I don't see my doll story as a lie. Surely I tell her what she wants to hear. But surely, living in our brand-new house and wearing our pretty clothes, we *are* happy. How can we not be? Since I am so happy, I'm not ordered to return to school. No authorities come to the house. No one investigates further.

Day after day I stay in my house. On sunny days my mother urges me outside. I sit on the front stoop, raking a stick through grass. I sit on the back stoop, tapping the stick on the brick patio. I leave the door ajar to hear my mother in case she calls to me. I glance inside the window where she sits on the couch reading the paper. I know she will leave me, I know she will die the moment I glance away. Still, she urges me farther from home. "Ride your bicycle," she tells me.

My muscles strain as I pedal up the steepest hill in the neighborhood. At the top I pause, one foot on the ground, my arms resting on the handlebar. The streets are deserted. All the fathers are in the city, working. All the kids are in school. Mothers wash breakfast dishes and straighten beds. Drowsy infants and toddlers are napping.

No birds call out to the sun. No leaves on trees rearrange the air. No squirrels dig holes in the ground to hide nuts for winter. No curtains flutter in windows. It is too warm for smoke to curl from chimneys. Clouds seem suspended in a flat, blue sky. There is no motion in any of the houses. Why are the houses so silent? Why can't I hear any voices? Or are there no voices because there is no one to hear mine? Right now I want someone to hear it. Everyone to hear it. Right now I feel like running the length of the street, beating at all the doors with a stick, beating and screaming: *Open up, open up—for me.*

I don't move. Still, the neighborhood is silent. In this absence of sound I think I hear a warning. Because of the utter stillness of this moment I can now hear. I glance around. What is the warning? Where is it? What does it want from me?

At the bottom of the hill, there, nestled beside the woods, is our pretty house, our neat yard, my father's work shed. From the outside, the shed looks quiet and peaceful, too. Yet inside is my father's electric saw. Sometimes when he uses it, even when I'm in the house, I think I feel the windows vibrate against my fingertips and the floorboards beneath my feet. And for this moment as I pause on top of the hill, in this stillness, I believe I hear, faintly at first, then louder, the whir of my father's saw turning, the silver blade spinning. But it is my body there—not a plank or a piece of plywood but rather my body clamped in the vise, my shoulder blades pressed against metal. And I must speed to it, to my body, save it—*this* is the warning—and I am speeding, quickly, quickly, back down the hill. Wands of sunlight reflect off the handlebar, circles of light spin in spokes of bicycle wheels, as I rush toward the shed, rush toward my body. But before I reach it . . .

I see the parked car clearly. There is no distracting traffic. There are no dogs, no children, no sudden noises. Only circles and circles of silver light wheeling down the pavement. And I must crash. I must. I crash into a parked car, crumpling my bike, shredding skin off my face.

Light hurts my face. So now, while I'm healing, I'm allowed to stay in the house with curtains drawn. This is what I wanted: to hide inside, behind curtains, where no one can smell the leakage from my body; to be safe inside, behind curtains, where I can be close to my body clamped to my father's electric saw. Besides, I am now able to weight the house with my constant presence. Otherwise, gravity would loosen its grip and the house would float away. I wouldn't be able to bear losing my house and my family, for I believe I am overwhelmingly loved by this family. Camp is bad, school is bad, not my home or my family. After all, my father holds me on his lap, my face against his undershirt, and strokes my hair. My parents buy me pretty dresses. My mother cooks us dinner and wears beautiful red lipstick. My father shows me his love, over and over, when he teaches me new things.

I am addicted to these terrifying new things. Addicted to terror. For terror, feel love. With terror, my body feels loved. Terror is the definition of love, a synonym proving love's existence. So I stubbornly sit in this house in order to enable my parents to love me. I need for my father to love me. And I believe that he does.

□ □ □

Night after night in the bathtub I watch my rubber duck. Its round rubber eyes watch me, too, for it is the first to see. Bits of scum float on the murky surface of water, and I believe it is pieces of skin scaled from my body. Perhaps I am losing bits of skin, parts of my body. Soon, perhaps, there will be nothing left. I don't look down at my daddy's hand. I don't look down at my body. I don't move. Not a finger. Not a toe. I'm not aware of breathing. But his breath—*his*—rushes. This is the only sound, this, I feel his breath as it rushes toward me across the water. There is no other sound in the house, none outside the white wood door of the bathroom. No one will enter; I know this. No one will knock on the door. Night after night my daddy bathes me and no one knocks. No one touches the knob. No one ever will. Even if someone did enter, what could she see in the steamy mirror, in the misty room that is underwater wet? Days. Weeks. Months. His rubbing grows more insistent. Soon small bubbles of panic rise in the water, and the duck jerks away in a fierce ripple of tides.

I close my eyes. I feel the skin of my eyes slip far far back in my skull. As his finger penetrates deep, deeper, I no longer have eyes. I no longer have my body. It is Dina, Dina, Dina. *You do it, Dina,* I say to her, in a voice only I can hear. *You do it. You want this. You, Dina, with your straight black hair, olive-colored skin, and the blackest of eyes.* It is her legs parted like that with his finger inside her . . . while I disappear in a bubble of water. Concentrate on the bubbles of water. They make soft explosions as they crash against the surface, but then another rise rise rises out the roof of my head. But the room is still, yes. I am. My legs are paralyzed. My arms are useless. I am bloated with hot, heavy water, yet weightless, too: here, not here. I am opposites at the same time. And from the distance of my bubble my hazel eyes watch my daddy stick his finger inside Dina, telling her, whispering to her how much he loves her—me—us, loves her—me—us, with a love that is everlasting and true.

□ □ □

I hide inside bubbles. I hide inside words, in my own invented words that soothe, in my own vocabulary, my own language, for surely my parents teach me no words that are useful. I soar on magical carpets woven with silken words and images that no one else understands. For example, when I learn the alphabet, it is not this endless string of anonymous letters that interests me. In particular, I never hear the individual letters *L, M, N, O.* Rather, to me these letters slur together to form the imaginary word "elimeno," really more image than true language. It is this magically real image—landing smack in the middle of *A* through *Z*—that interrupts the droning litany of the one-after-another letters.

The image "elimeno" is a school of elementary minnows darting through cool pools of water, weaving around undulating grasses in the lap-lap of the sea. I believe the minnows swim to elementary school, swimming past coral reefs the color of fire and opals, their bodies glittering like sun shafts deep in the sea.

Then, like turning a kaleidoscope, as the beauty of this image fades, "elimeno" is magically transformed into a gorgeous yellow lemon. Now it is this taste in my mouth, this sunny summery taste of puckered lemonyellow, this taste, no other, as if "lemonyellow" is the only word I need ever know. The only word I want ever to taste. So when I'm in the bathtub—no—I'm not there: I'm in the sea with minnows; and when I taste something else in my mouth—no—it vanishes, replaced with a sunny lemon taste. And then I live—I am so lucky to live in the most beautiful place in the world.

□ □ □

There is one home I visit in the neighborhood. There is one person I want to see, although she's barely a person yet, just the smallest of babies. For hours I sit next to Beth's crib. Pale eyelashes of her sleeping eyes form half-moons on the lids. Sunlight burnishes her wispy, gold-red hair and sometimes I whisper my fingers through it like a comb, careful not to tug it. Saliva bubbles her tiny lips and baby powder clumps in creases of elbows and knees and toes. Sometimes I worry who will wipe the saliva and who will clean the creases. I worry her diapers need changing. I worry her body needs bathing. I worry about who will change them and who will bathe her. I want to be able to watch her endlessly, never take my eyes off her, although I don't understand this need. She opens her eyes. I smile, my face pressed against the bars of the crib. She gurgles and coos. Do I wonder who you are? Do I wonder if I were ever a baby like you?

□ □ □

When officials from the Trust Territories are in town, they dine with us at the house: Governors Paul McNutt of the Philippines, Oren Long of Hawaii, Ernest Gruening of Alaska, Luis Muñoz-Marin of Puerto Rico, Phelps Phelps of Samoa, Morris de Castro of the Virgin Islands. My daddy and I greet our company at the door while my mother cooks in the kitchen. I wear frilly dresses with white socks and patent-leather shoes. I offer hors d'oeuvres arranged on monkeypod platters and carry drinks in white linen cocktail napkins. I smile. I sing songs. I love to show off my dolls. I am a beloved pet performing, showing what a happy child I am, what a happy family we are.

After everyone leaves, the house again is quiet. No, it is more than quiet. Where is my sister? I never know. I stand in the living room in my pretty dress staring out the picture window into the nighttime yard. But I see no yard. In the glass the living room is reflected, so there is no outside world at all: no yard, no trees, nothing beyond that window. And I—all of us—are trapped inside the glass, for even if my sister fled the house, her flight, her need for flight, is the trap itself. And inside the house, if I scream, no one will hear. If I could scream, I know that glass would shatter.

But my father is the only one with a voice, the only one who knows how to scream. If something went wrong during the party . . . if the food were not perfect . . . if some detail were overlooked, then, after everyone leaves, his rage is swift and solid. But the glass on the window will never shatter, for his wrath is turned on us, his three little girls. It is our brittle bones that will absorb the shock of his voice. We are the only ones who will ever hear him, for everyone outside the house believes my father is perfect. In the midst of his anger, my mother will cry. I will cry. My sister will be dry and vacant. I wait to be hit. If I am, then later, while my mother washes dishes, my father and I go down the hall to the bathroom, to the bathtub, where he loves to soothe me. Perhaps I am almost asleep by the time he undresses me and slips me into the water. His voice whispers that he adores me, that all he wants is to make me happy. "Suzie, my most precious daughter. You are more precious to me than life," he tells me, while his finger, ever so gently, enters my drowsy body.

□ □ □

I wake in the middle of the night. It is quiet. I am alone—but not quiet. Earlier, my mother had told me stories about her war, a war that, even though she didn't experience it directly, haunts her. That song about Hitler is not all she's taught me. So I am restless, unable to sleep. I lie in bed gazing out the high windows in my room. But all I can see are the thousands of yellow stars once sewn on clothes of Jewish children, marking them, identifying them. I wonder why parents hadn't ripped off the stars and transformed their children with costumes and masks.

□ □ □

When Eisenhower is elected President, my father loses his position with the government. He stays home, inside the house, unable to leave the house for weeks. Without a job he must be very frightened, although my mother claims—to friends, to neighbors, to her daughters—that he suffers from pneumonia. Since I am still home from school, I am assigned to care for him. We are truant together.

My father lies in bed day after day, week after week, in a dark bedroom, the curtains drawn. I also close the raw silk curtains in the living room, believing darkness is comforting and will heal my father back to health. I spoon-feed him soup for lunch. I nudge saltine crackers against his mouth. I hold a straw for him to drink liquids. His stillness scares me. I am scared he will die and that somehow, if he does, all three of his girls will die with him.

My mother drifts in and out of my consciousness, in and out of the house. She goes shopping. She visits neighbors. My sister bangs into the house after school, changes her clothes, bangs outside again to play with friends. But let her go, I think. I don't care. My father will love me more because I'm the good girl who stays with him, even better than my mother. I will care for him until he is well. I am the only one who can cure him.

Evening wilts over the eaves of the house. I hear my mother in the kitchen fixing dinner. I sit in the bedroom with my father. No, I am not sitting in the bedroom with my father. I am lying in bed next to him. He holds up the sheet and motions me to get under the covers. He presses me close, and I believe my body itself can nurse him back to health. He takes my hand and slips it inside his boxer shorts and places it on this thing. I don't know what it is; it must be swelling caused by pneumonia. It must be, but it is hard and scary and all I want is for him to be well soon, for the swelling to go down. As he guides my hand, I fall farther and farther into the darkness of the room, sheets lowering over us like banks of clouds descending. Until I am jolted back—when the sickness of this swelling erupts all over my hand. The suddenness of it on my hand—and I . . . I think it is blood and pus, that he is bleeding to death, that I have caused it to bleed, and I scream, once, for my mother, struggling with sheets, trying to run to the kitchen for my mother, before he slaps me across the mouth with such force my head cracks against the headboard. And I am stunned, forever, into silence.

My mother doesn't come; she must not have heard me. But soon I am okay. His loving words return, so I know he's not dying, that

I haven't done anything to kill him. He tells me I am his precious, his only precious, that I am healing my daddy, that my mommy doesn't know how to do this, that I am the only one in the world who will make daddy better, and now I must lick my hand clean, lick him clean, that my beautiful, beautiful tongue can heal him—haven't I seen cats lick their kittens?—and when I finish he kisses me on my mouth, but no, it is Dina who licks us clean, Dina who loves my father without question, Dina who opens her mouth, the way he teaches us, and Dina is the best pupil.

While he is sick we spend hours together. When my mother is home I'm in my clothes, sitting on a chair or on the edge of the bed. Only when she leaves can I truly begin to cure him. *No, you, Dina, you heal him.* In the movement of her head nodding, I become a glimmer of light on the darkest pane of glass. Watching Dina in bed with my father, I am a mote of dust or a ripple in the bedroom curtain. When he whispers he loves her, she whispers back. He caresses her body. He teaches her to let him put his mouth and tongue between her legs, teaches her how to put her mouth where he is sick, on the swelling. But why is it that after Dina finishes, why is it that after, it is my mouth that tastes this? Why is it that my jaw feels weary, and not Dina's? I am angry at Dina for not doing a better job. *You will do a better job*, I rage at her. *You will not leave me with this mess to clean up, it is your mess to clean up—it isn't mine.* I put gobs of toothpaste in my mouth. But every time I swallow, I taste it.

I have disappeared. No one knows where I am. I sit in a tiny cupboard, but even I don't know where I am, which room I hide in. I'm not even sure whether I'm hiding or whether I'm merely lost. I don't know how long I've been here or how I came to be here, why I'm here. The only connection I have to that which is outside the cupboard is a crack of light surrounding the cupboard door. I hear my mother's voice calling, but I don't know my name and there is no voice with which to answer. I feel nothing. There is no cramp in my legs, even though I am hunched tight. I don't even feel as if I have legs. I don't know whether I wear clothes or not. The smell of my body overpowers all other senses.

Finally the door is yanked open. I am yanked out. My legs buckle and I slide onto the floor—the bathroom floor—this is where I am, in blinding light. I wear only an undershirt and blood is smudged on my thighs. *No, no, look more closely: The blood is between your thighs, you, Dina, between your disgusting, filthy thighs. No wonder your mother must slap you, slap you, scream at you, you, your mother must call you disgusting, you bad, bad girl, what did you do to yourself, you slutslutslut.* But neither Dina nor I can answer her; we don't understand the source of the blood. In our silence, she fills the tub with water and throws us in. *No, you Dina, she throws you in, her hand rough, rough, scrubbing you between your legs, that disgusting place.* She scrubs and scrubs and scrubs, first with her sharp fingers, then with a white terry washcloth until *you burn, asking you what you did to yourself, telling you, screaming at you, you slut. No man will marry you. Men don't marry sluts.*

I watch slow swirls of blood tint the water. I am this blood. And I know I will drown.

She throws the washcloth in the garbage and empties the water. She tells me to put my feet on opposite sides of the tub, and she inserts a rubber nozzle attached to our enema bottle into that spot. She will clean this dirty, disgusting slut inside and out. She has mixed something in the bottle and I am relieved, for I know my body needs a potion stronger than water, perhaps an astringent, in order to clean it well. At first it stings. I feel a deep burn pulsing through me. Soon I become the burning itself; there is no difference. I want to be. My body needs to be cleansed with, as much as I need to become, white hot heat. And I am no longer a body.

Afterwards our house is rigid. I am rigid. Rigidly, we cook and clean, speak and eat. My legs are the most rigid of all. My breaths are short and shallow, my steps small. Every time I move I believe I rip out all the stitches that hold my body together.

□ □ □

The curtains in the house are open. My father gets out of bed. He is to open a bank in St. Thomas with Congressman Fred Crawford, and we will all move to the tropics. With this news I feel released. My father is no longer sick. He leaves the house. A siege has ended. That swelling on his body must have gone down.

I even go outside, wander in the woods behind our house. In the early winter a few gold and red leaves still cling to trees. I gather fallen leaves from the ground and press them to my face: They smell of woodsmoke, of deep burgundy, of last traces of sunlight as well as the first white scent of winter. The leaves feel fragile and smell as cool as the ground. These scents seem new; I don't remember smelling them before. And now I won't see autumn again for a long time. Yet while it's peaceful here, and beautiful, I am not nostalgic. I want to move. I believe that who we are here, who I am here, will be left behind; we will be new people in the tropics. My father won't catch pneumonia again in the warm, peaceful tropics.

A creek winds through the woods. Low bushes and branches drip. This is all—there are no voices, no calls from birds—only the sound of water rushing, this gray scent of riverwater. I hover on the bank, the warmth of sun-reflected water brushing my legs, and watch the current swirling around a large rock in the middle of the creek. What power, I think, that the rock can interrupt the flow of water of the fast-moving stream.

Then I know it isn't water that draws me. For I'm afraid of water, afraid of what is hidden below the surface. Rather, I'm drawn to the rock. I want to sit on it. By leaping from stone to stone I near it, careful the water not touch me.

Above the water the rock is warm. I lie on it and feel this warmth slowly seep through my body. I press my ear to the surface, listening until I hear the sound of water throbbing rock. Except—I know what I must truly be hearing is the sound of the rock's heartbeat, beating safely, beating strongly, protected deep inside solid layers of stone. I listen and listen, as if I can learn this secret language of rock, the only sound I want to be able to hear. I listen until, yes, I hear my own heartbeat throbbing, my own heart beat, safely hidden deep inside the rock.

□ □ □

A letter addressed to my mother on Kingswood Road in Bethesda, from my father, who is in St. Thomas. It is dated October 29, 1954—their anniversary:

> Dear Precious Ketzie,
>
> We're separated again. I hope I can reach you by telephone tonight. I shall call you about 9:00.
>
> It's hard to believe that 21 years flew by so quickly. We've gone through so much together. There have been many heartaches and much grief, but each year we're brought closer and closer together. I guess the full and true significance of married life is not realized until the years roll-by. The com-

pleteness and oneness and the mysteriousness is not fully understood until the trials and tribulations mixed with untold joy and happiness are experienced year after year.

I wish so much that we were here both together on this day. I miss you more than I can say. I know that you understand even though you are hundreds of miles away. I love you so very very much.

All day long, events of the past years have been going through my mind: the train trip to N. Y.; the week on the Georgic; our trip to Europe; our arrival in Haifa; the first night; Passover at Zichron; our week in Jerusalem; the Bar Examination; our trip back on the Polonia; our trip back through Europe; our return to N. Y. and to Chicago by Bus; the episode in the Cleaning Business; my first job in Washington; 2131 "O" St.; our walks to work in the morning; the purchase of our first car; our trip to Mexico; moving to 3920 Southern Ave.; the job at the Library; meeting you at the open window; coming home that evening when you met me, wearing your brown coat, telling me that you were pregnant; the Friday when Kiki was born; the exhileration driving home that night after having seen Kiki for the first time; the war; my induction; then your walking down the steps going to Doctor's Hospital; Little Susie's coming; the building of our house and now here. So much has happened: it's hard to relive all the joy, the happiness and the bitterness and heartache as well.

Sweet precious. I wish so much you were here with me tonight. I feel so lonely and alone. I hope at least to be speaking with you in a few hours. Good night sweet precious. I love you and miss you so very very much.

Night Spirits

St. Thomas: 1953–1958

In St. Thomas we live in a Danish colonial house next to Blackbeard's Castle on Blackbeard's Hill. My bedroom is at one end of the house with three separate entrances. One can enter it from a wood porch which wraps around the mountain side of the house and overlooks the Caribbean. Or one can enter it from the stone terrace on the opposite side of the house, the land side, next to Blackbeard's Castle and a dead-end street. Or one can enter my bedroom through my sister's, although she keeps the door between our rooms shut tight.

The bed in which I sleep is mahogany, a four-poster with a mosquito net that drapes from ceiling to floor. At night, trade winds ruffle the Caribbean, skim the sea, then drift ashore to rustle the leaves of coconut palm and sea-grape trees before sweeping up the mountain to the porch door of my bedroom, trailing scents of the island and of the sea, and disturbing the marquisette netting over my bed before continuing their journey across savannahs and up volcanic mountains beyond.

From the start, I believe I belong on this tropical island in the Antilles, in the West Indies. This island—immutable, drowsy, swollen with heat—seems familiar. I also believe I belong at All-Saints

Parish, an Anglican school where I complete second grade. I must belong here because the religious rituals enchant me as much as I am enchanted by my images of the Egyptian princess. They transform me. Now I imagine the Egyptian princess is decorated with Christian symbols. My fingers grasp a garnet rosary. A cross hangs from my neck.

At school on Good Friday our foreheads are marked with charcoal. Even though all the children at school have identical crosses on their foreheads, I believe this mark distinguishes me. I believe mine is different. I am the Egyptian princess who has been specially chosen to soothe angry gods—not the other children. My Egyptian body, adorned with Christian amulets, is needed to end a drought, to enhance a bountiful harvest. My body has been selected to save Mankind. With this mark I am anointed. I want it branded into my skin. That night I refuse to wash the mark from my forehead. By morning the cross is a faint blur. I try to darken it with a pencil.

□ □ □

A few days after we arrive on the island, we learn many islanders believe that the bank my father has come here to open is for his gain, not for their own, as he claims. They organize a demonstration—a march from Market Square to Emancipation Park—to burn my father in effigy. He decides to go to the park to address the crowd and alleviate their fears. He will remind them that, while still with the government, he helped pass the Home Rule Bill for the Virgin Islands. He will tell them the next step toward economic independence for the islands is this bank, the West Indies Bank and

Trust Company. Before, blacks had kept their money at home, not earning interest, not receiving loans. My father's bank is to encourage tourism, to give loans to islanders who want to start small businesses, to sell stock to the islanders at low rates.

For protection during the demonstration, my sister and I are locked by ourselves in Riise's rum warehouse on Main Street, a thick brick and stucco building constructed to withstand hurricanes, fires, and pirates. My sister and I press our ears to the arched metal door. Shouts, the pound of drums echo against the walls. The smell of smoke seeps across the threshold. Through the keyhole I glimpse fiery torches. Nevertheless, I believe I would feel safer outside than in this massive warehouse, dimly lit by a few bulbs dangling from the high ceiling.

"Do you think they'll be okay?" my sister asks—meaning our parents. I stare at her, stunned, confused. I didn't know my sister felt fear. I nod, suddenly transformed into the older sister. "Of course," I say, nodding to reassure her, then not even afraid of the warehouse.

Soon there is silence; soon we grow tired. We wander to the rear of the warehouse, full of mahogany rum barrels. The sweet smell of rum and mahogany, the lingering scent of smoke, make us dizzy. We sit on the brick floor propped against a rum barrel.

"You want me to rub your back?" my sister asks. She knows I hate to have my back rubbed; rather, I know *she* is the one who finds it soothing.

"How about if I rub yours first," I say, knowing this is what she intended. She lies down, her face on my legs. My fingers trickle across her back, round and around. My legs go to sleep, my arm is cramped, but I continue, not wanting to lose my sister. If I stop she'll pull away from me, and I love my sister.

Later, in the distance, I hear cheering. Of course my father is a hero. His bank will be a success. Most who know my father respect and admire him. I am proud of him. He is *my* father. I am grateful for how much he loves me.

□ □ □

Almost every night my parents dine at the Virgin Isle Hotel, entertaining potential investors for the island. While it is now possible for me to be away from my mother during the day, this is not true for night. The more nights I am scared by night, the more nights I need her, need her to protect me from it. I don't want her to go. Dusk in the West Indies is fleeting and as soon as the sun sets, the fear begins. So to try to keep my mother from leaving me, I throw myself against the wall, I scratch myself, I cry. She can't console me. She rushes out the door behind my father and doesn't hear me say good-bye.

After their car drives down the mountain, I silently lie on my bed, listening, waiting. The folds in the mosquito net cast shadows. At the base of the mountain, I believe I hear the murmur of waves. I close my eyes. I know what will soon come. For even though I seem to be alone, I am not. Now, just past dusk, it is the moment, it is the time, when the sighs and tremors of Caribbean spirits begin. Some spirits are as gentle as white petals of ginger flowers. Others are as dark as a long Caribbean night. For at night these dangerous spirits extinguish the sun, cloak the moon, snuff out the stars, veil the sky. This is when, if I'm not careful, these spirits—with their red-red mouths and whispering fingers—might discover my drowsing body. So every night I must believe, truly believe, my body is swaddled in soft ginger and hibiscus petals, slowly curling inward for night, protecting me from dark spirits of night.

Later, much later, my restless body senses my parents driving back up the mountain. Even in slumber my body snuggles deeper inside its petaled armor.

□ □ □

For third grade I transfer to the Antilles School. After school I take the bus to town. There, I either wait for my father to drive me up the mountain or else I, like my sister, begin to wander the island, drifting farther from home. I explore fields of guinea grass and royal poinciana trees. Sometimes I attend movies at the Center Theatre. I see *The House of Wax*, *Mojave Firebrand*, *The Man with the Steel Whip*, *Fury of the Congo*.

Other afternoons I play with my friends, kids of different ages from the Antilles or All-Saints Parish schools. Patti, with silky red hair and blue eyes, lives with her divorced mother. Always, there are whispered rumors about her mother and married men, and dust from these rumors seems to settle on Patti as if she is as involved with these men as her mother. When I spend the night with Patti, we trail our fingers across black negligees, red slips, lacy bras found in her mother's dresser. We inhale the scent of mimosa and frangipani perfume and decorate our faces with crimson lipstick and violet eye shadow. I don't associate these colors or scents of sex with my father. In fact, if asked what I know about sex, I would blush and say, "Nothing." To me, this would not be a lie. I never define my relationship with my father. The secret we share is given no word. I would never have called it "sex." To me, *this* would be the lie.

Maria's house hides other secrets—hides her mother, who drinks silently, seldom leaving the house; hides her father, who, when he drinks, beats his children. Maria and Mike, her brother, shrug off their bruises. I know Maria from All-Saints Parish School, and when I spend the night with her, her mother, whom I see only at prayers, makes us pray on our knees before sleeping. The room is in dark green shadows. Her mother smells of incense, of rum, of sleep. In low voices we mumble "if I should die before I wake . . ." I believe this could be true.

Inga and I spend hours reading on her cool stone veranda. I hear the rustle of lizards, the turning of pages, the flutter of dove wings in the bushes. Inga tests our reading skills to determine who can read the most pages in ten minutes. She always beats me, except when I cheat, turning two pages at a time, feeling a need to win, to beat this girl who seems perfect with her curly blonde hair and her silent home, a silence that reflects the cool, frosty blue of her eyes. I crave this cool, this frost, and dread the moment her mother drives me home. Sometimes I stay for dinner. We eat in a formal dining room with a large mahogany table, a table set with blue Wedgwood plates and cut crystal. Her father wears a dinner jacket and bow tie; her mother, spotless, unwrinkled linen. She tinkles a small glass bell when the maid is to serve platters of food around the table. If her father doesn't like the food, he makes no mention of it.

My friends and I meet in the deep curve of horseshoe-shaped Magens Bay. Maria and I chew bitter sea grapes and dribble wet sand into castles. Inga lies on a towel, reading. Patti, in her red suit, stares out to sea, watching for the *Danmark,* a training ship of young Danish sailors. Every year it sails into port, and every year a dance is held with local schoolgirls. We are too young to go, but still Patti waits. Not far from shore, Skip and Billy splash and toss a beach ball.

Late in the afternoon we explore the rocky peninsula jutting into the sea. Spindrifts crash against limestone boulders, spraying us with salty water. Sunlight skates across the lavender, azure, turquoise surface of the sea. Although we move slowly, mindful of sea urchins hiding in shallow tidepools, I pretend I am racing toward the horizon, that I've just spied a pirate ship—Blackbeard—his galleon skimming the waves. I am marooned—no one can find me—he has come searching for me, to rescue me. I call to him. I beckon. Even from here I see sunlight glancing off the ruby earring he wears in the lobe of his ear. His gold sword sparkles. And I will sail away with him in his galleon, with the scent of rum, with wind smacking the sails. Climbing these rocks, in the shadow of towering mountain peaks, I do not notice the endless, deserted horizon, the empty, empty sea.

Soon dusk slides from these mountaintops into this sea. The sun punctures the water. We glance toward shore, by now almost too tired to trek back on rocks that are slippery and uneven. We are too hot, too thirsty. No one has remembered to bring fresh water. We are ill-prepared in the nurturing and nourishment of our bodies. When we finally reach our towels we are angry and sullen, too exhausted to speak. Always, I believe my friends suffer from the same exhaustion as I. Always, I am disappointed no pirate has sailed to the island for me, that I will not wield a gold sword or wear a ruby earring in the lobe of one ear. I will not feel thick hemp rope in my calloused hands. These images are neither fantasy nor daydream. This habitat of truthful magic is where I live. It is a secret that is mine.

□ □ □

The Antilles School is high on a mountain. Its veranda and classrooms overlook the entrance to the harbor, drenched in tropical sunlight. White sails billow. Seagulls wing across the blue vault of sky. I am restless. School is boring. While I want to concentrate, I can't. I have trouble listening in school, for these are not the voices I want to hear. I gaze out paneless windows until this magical power I possess finally gusts me outside and I am flowing into newly discovered scents and sounds of the West Indies. The flutter of hummingbird wings. The drip of frangipani leaves after a tropical rain. This soothing language is one I believe belongs only to me. I am with these scents, of these sounds, while able to leave my dull, dull body far behind.

Yet I wonder: Is this body alone or is it with Dina's? If it's with Dina, are two bodies actually present? Sometimes I feel as if strands of her black hair are braided tight with my own. She must know what I do; I know what she does. Even so, we aren't the same. There is a difference. For at other times our hair unravels and we are attached by the thinnest of membranes. It unravels at night—when *she* is the one who waits for my father—while I grasp filaments of a spiderweb and climb a silken ladder to the most distant planet or star. These are the times I'm able to watch her from a distance, the times I don't have her feelings, the times her experiences don't have to be mine.

So who is it—Dina or me—this afternoon on the school veranda? I've been the one playing volleyball, and I am the one now holding a white paper cup, waiting in line with my friends at the bubbler. We are allowed only one cup of water, far from enough, and I am the one who is thirsty. Now, on this particular day, I am also exhausted from heat and faint after finishing my water.

At first, upon waking, I feel the cement floor beneath my legs. Then I hear the voice of the school handyman, a black man, fanning me with a palm-leaf fan and offering me a second cup of water. Through the thin paper cup I feel the cool water against my fingertips. I am so grateful I'm almost afraid to drink it, not wanting, ever, to finish it.

"Go on," he tells me. "It's for you. Drink it."

I do, and after I finish he helps me to the far end of the veranda, where I sit at a table to rest.

Two older boys come and sit across from me. Tough, sullen, they say, "You let that native man see down your blouse, but you don't let us, you know what they'll say about you?"

I recognize something familiar in their eyes and I know I am not supposed to answer.

"Nigger lover," they say.

I collapse the paper cup in my fist and stare at it. They laugh at me and say: "Nigger lover, nigger lover, suck your nigger titty. You let us look, we won't tell anyone what we saw that nigger do."

Of course I know nothing happened while I fainted. Even without looking I know my jumper is safely snapped. But I have this fear I'll never be able to speak again or explain anything. So when they tell me to lean under the table, I do. They unsnap my jumper and stare at my flat child breasts. At first they laugh nervously, but then they simply stare. They don't touch me.

It is now that I know—this is the moment—I am no longer me. Slowly, almost imperceptibly, my hazel eyes fade into Dina's black ones. It is Dina's gaze that shamefully turns from the boys to blankly watch the ground.

The headmistress catches us—catches me. I am ordered to the bathroom, where she washes my mouth with soap. She calls to tell my mother. When I get home my mother takes off my pants and hits me with a belt, but by this time I know she is right, know my body deserves to be punished. I believe everything she says about my body is true. I expect to be punished. I relish it, even believe that with her strikes my body is purified. I believe my mother is the only one capable of cleansing my body.

My mother tells my father: Sue was caught showing her breasts to the boys at school.

His jealousy shows me how much he loves me. That night he bites my nipples until they bleed, tells me they belong to him, that I am never to let another man see them or touch them, that he will kill me next time, that he can make my body into a body no man would ever be able to stand to look at. My body can only be his.

Yes, Daddy, I believe you, for I know it could never be mine.

He is right. For in the heat of St. Thomas my father, too, is thirsty. He, too, doesn't have enough to drink, so he must drink my sweat, my blood, my saliva. He must drink and drink and drink.

□ □ □

My mother throws a pair of my white cotton underpants at my feet. There is a stain on them, she says, and she will not give them to our maid, Sylvanita, to wash. She would be embarrassed. I should be embarrassed. She orders me to wash them until every trace of stain is removed. We have no hot water in St. Thomas, and I stand at the bathroom sink for over an hour scrubbing with cold water. The bar of soap melts to a nub. My legs ache from standing. My fingers are numb. I don't know what the stain is. It is slightly yellow, murky, a shameful leakage, an evil discharge from my body—no, Dina's body, I tell myself. And I know my mother is right that it must be removed.

At dinnertime my mother checks on me. I show her the progress—really there is none—and I'm told I will wear these underpants to dinner, that we don't have money to be buying new underpants. Throughout dinner I sit in cold wet pants. I don't know if she has told my father or my sister, but I am too ashamed to eat. Too exhausted. My father is the only one who ever talks at dinner, telling us about his day, his work, his career. No one listens. Surely, we all are too tired. We are all, in our different ways, all of us, worn to a nub.

Soon afterward my back begins to hurt. It feels like a weight, as if my lower back is too swollen to move. I believe it is permanently chilled from the wet underpants.

□ □ □

In fourth grade a new teacher comes to the school, an Englishman, Mr. Gerrard. Since St. Thomas was owned by Denmark before being bought by the United States, there are no British accents, and we are not tolerant of his differentness. Besides, his body smells sour, and he is, in the opinion of my class, quite homely. We tease him mercilessly. We disrupt class. We hold our noses when he walks by. We laugh at him. We ignore his authority as a teacher. Surely it is upon this man, this lonely stranger, that I act out the rage my family deserves. I sense the vulnerability of a newcomer, sense his timidity. I have learned the art of being a predator from my parents. Surely he receives the wrath that is nightly implanted into my body. I scorn his weakness—not wanting to see my own in him. My classmates and I shame him from the island in less than a year. But I am the one who is truly, forever, shamed.

□ □ □

One evening when my father is in the States on business, my mother spends hours helping me memorize the multiplication tables. 4×7? 8×3? 6×7? I don't know, I don't know, I don't know. The hour grows later. I manage to remember a few correct answers, but I am far away from knowing them all. For a while I stand on my head, thinking the extra blood in my brain will help my memory. Then I climb a doorway, a trick I learned from my sister. By putting a foot on either side of the wide jambs, with palms also pressed to the jambs, I shinny up to the top, quite high, as the ceilings are high. Maybe I can think better from up here. I can't. I slide halfway down, then jump, waking our dachshund, Oscar. He begins to bark and we put him out on the porch. 7×9? Sevens are the worst. My mother keeps drilling me, and it is close to midnight when we become hysterical. Soon we are laughing so hard we're crying, she as hard as I. I will never learn these numbers; I will never be able to stop laughing; I will never be able to stop crying. Oscar continues to bark. No one in my family will ever be able to stop.

□ □ □

My mother receives the following letter from my father, still in the States on business:

Dear Precious,

I have your long letter. I am very sorry you were hurt about my asking Morris to hold all the mail for me. I did tell him specifically only to hold the office mail—to give you all other mail. I told him to do so because heretofore I found on my return all the mail which had accumulated during my absence strewn all over my desk as well as in the box on my desk. I never know who in my absence is looking at the mail and there might be letters which arrived in my absence which I did not find. I therefore asked Morris to be sure to keep all the mail for me, that is official mail until I returned. I am sorry that was misunderstood and I am sorry that it added to your troubles. I have no secrets and you know that I do not have any. There is nothing that I need hide from you.

I write a letter to my daddy:

How are you? I am just beautiful, darling. I'd like you to bring me a string of blue popit beads, and I would like the smallest size bead there is and a long string of the beads. Is it cold up there? did it snow? We took our dancing lesson today, it was good. We got Oscar a new collar. Oscar sends his love.

□ □ □

Maria looks pretty for her birthday party, wearing a white dress with crinolines. A white hibiscus is pinned in her short dark hair. I place my present on the table and sit beside her, waiting for the others to arrive. Sandwiches, crusts trimmed from the sides, are on china platters surrounding a birthday cake with white icing and pink roses. Coke and 7-Up bubble in crystal glasses. The maid has prepared this food and set the table before going home. Maria's mother will be in her room, drinking. Her father? Maria shakes her head. Mike, her brother, has eaten one of the pink roses off the cake and her father is punishing him. Her brother has been taken to his room.

Even after the kids arrive I sit beside the table. I notice the spot where her eight-year-old brother plucked the pink rose neatly from its nest of white icing. But since I believe he surely hasn't eaten enough, I decide I must bring him another piece of cake. I cut a huge slice from another corner, where there are two roses, and wrap it in a napkin.

I slip away, carrying the cake in both hands. Inside the house, my buffalo-hide sandals slap across the vertivert rugs on the wood floor of the living room. Slowly I climb the stairs to the second story. All the doors off the hall are shut. Behind the door of her parents' bedroom, her mother sits with closed hurricane shutters. I wonder if she knows there's a party; I wonder if she knows it's her daughter's birthday.

I want to race down the hall, banging on doors and shouting. I want to wake up this house. But I creep silently. I will make no sound. I feel light, as thin as air, and I believe myself invisible. I must not get caught, because if I do, the cake will be taken away and I must feed Mike more cake. When I reach his shut door I'm afraid to set the cake on the floor, afraid to relinquish it for even a moment, so I hold it against my chest, even though it's getting squashed. With my other hand I turn the glass knob. The door gives. I push it inch by inch, feeling warm air seep toward me over the threshold. The room is dim. A ceiling fan barely stirs sweaty air. Mike lies on his bed, on his stomach. His back has been cut by a tamarind switch that is now in the corner. I sit beside him. He doesn't open his eyes.

I break off a small piece of cake and press it to his mouth. Nothing happens. I don't move, just wait, wait for him to smell it, wait for him to understand it is for him, and it is all right for him to eat it. When his lips finally part and my fingers nudge the cake inside, he waits a moment before chewing. As soon as he swallows, I break off another piece, then another. He chews faster now, not once opening his eyes. When he is finished, I let him lick my fingers to soothe him, because I'm worried he is still hungry. I want to feed him more and more, fill him, nourish him, nurture him with food.

□ □ □

The Virgin Isle Hotel looks like a gigantic white bird nesting atop a volcanic mountain. The hotel is owned by Billy's family, and on Sundays he and I swim in the turquoise pool until the skin on my fingers puckers. After, we lounge on the terrace sunning ourselves while waiters bring us hamburgers, chocolate milk shakes, and Cokes. No one monitors us or asks for money. Billy simply signs the check. We play Hide and Seek down corridors and along terraces, in the cool marble lobby, behind cabanas. Sometimes we enter the woods, breathless, sweaty, but young, safe with each other. In the distance a donkey brays. Mongooses scurry in the undergrowth. I hide behind mimosa and royal poinciana trees, waiting for him to find me. When he does, we laugh. His skin smells of limes and the sun. And I want . . . I never want to lose his smell of limes, I never want to lose it, and don't understand the urgency to stay with him here in the woods, to make his smell, just by playing games with him, mine.

But later, tired from the afternoon sun, we sit in the Foolish Virgin Bar. Fish nets, filled with green and blue glass floats, hang from the ceiling. We order ginger ale and bowls of maraschino cherries and peanuts. I alternate—cherries and peanuts, cherries and peanuts, sweet and salt—until my lips and fingers are stained red and dotted white with salt. I stay with Billy until dusk, when we lean against the wrought-iron rail surrounding the terrace and watch the sun, the color of a crimson hibiscus, stain the Caribbean red. Far below, ships in the harbor rock in currents. The mound of bauxite on the pier darkens. The massive volcanic mountains seem thicker, more opaque, in evening darkness. Soon Charlotte Amalie, below us, is sprinkled with lights. Stars spike the sky. Then Billy leaves for home. I watch him go. It is time for me to meet my parents and my sister for dinner.

For dinner, at the hotel, tables are set with white cloths and polished silver. Magenta and yellow tropical flowers scent the room. Men wear white linen jackets and women in elegant gowns smell of expensive French perfume. The wooden dance floor gleams. The steel-drum band, wearing calypso shirts, plays on a raised stage. There will be a show. Usually professionals teach tourists how to dance the calypso, the merengue, the limbo.

Later, my father and I dance together. I am crisp and starched, my skirt bouyed with crinolines, my patent-leather shoes shining. Rarely does he dance with my mother, and never with my sister. We twirl around. He holds me tight and I smell his bay rum aftershave. Everyone smiles at us, dancing. I am a good dancer and everyone thinks I'm cute—this young girl dancing with her father. And later still, much later, this scent of bay rum will be on my skin, on Dina's body. But while we dance I wonder what my mother thinks. *Are you jealous, Mother? Are you hurt? Or maybe you're relieved, relieved to have relinquished your duties as wife to your daughter.*

□ □ □

Always, my mother kisses me good-night, tucking the marquisette net under the mattress to protect me while I sleep. Then the shudder of net as my father opens the door leading from the porch, the quiver of net as he gently untucks it and slips onto my white sheets.

I am always the lover he seeks on his nightly journey to my bed, too far away from his own. He kisses me and eases off my underpants and nightgown. He decorates my body with strand after strand of blue beads. He caresses my body, wanting me to love what he does as much as he loves it, wanting my body to desire his body—now, right now, when he can no longer delay, when he must enter me, when he can no longer wait. Except sometimes, these moments, he must notice my true-true body: cool as granite; rigid as rage. With incomprehension, lost in his own rage, desperately needing just one part of my body more than he needs sanity or love, he begins to hurt me . . . unless . . . quickly, quickly I metamorphose. Quickly silky black hair whispers across my shoulders and quickly I offer him Dina. Dina, whose body supplicates, whose body desires. Dina, who will be his childlover forever, his nightdaughter, whose body is never cool, never granite. I give my daddy the gift of Dina. Dina. Dina. Never, even once, will she refuse.

□ □ □

At the outdoor market I buy a slice of sugarcane and examine crates of papaya, mango, pineapple, plantains. I sit on an old rum barrel and dig my teeth into yellow, pulpy cane and chew it until only the skin remains. In my red French madras playsuit and buffalo-hide sandals, I am an island girl wandering through town. At Katz's Pharmacy I, along with other patrons, tap dimes on the counter until we are waited on. I buy a scoop of chocolate ice cream from Mr. Katz's daughter, several years older than I. Her eyes are lined with black and she wears her long ponytail braided. She is beautiful. I decide to braid my ponytail as well. I explore shady, brick-lined alleys of Beretta Center, where duty-free shops sell jewelry, perfume, Sea Isle cotton, cashmere sweaters, Madeira linens, doeskin cloth, French madras dresses, carnation and lavender Morny soap, West Indian rum. I follow tourists and wonder what it would be like if they took me home. I linger in front of Mr. Beretta's jewelry store, gazing at rows of amethysts, emeralds, diamonds, rubies, sapphires, pearls. I want to hold these cool, smooth jewels in my hands. My sister is inside with Mr. Beretta, sprawled on a wicker chair as if she's been there for hours. My sister always spends more time with acquaintances than with anyone who might grow close to her. She knows the shopkeepers far better than I, and one day Mr. Beretta gives her a ruby ring, her birthstone. Then, perhaps as an afterthought, he gives me a diamond ring, my birthstone, in the shape of a flower.

I visit Little Switzerland, next to my father's bank. It is the only place on the island with air-conditioning, and I love the blast of cold as I enter. I wander aisles of Wedgwood, silverware, watches, cuckoo clocks. All the jewelry, all the bottles of rum and liquor, all the imported tablecloths, all the perfumes soothe me. I am soothed by the cool perfection of cut gems. I am soothed by perfect-ticking Swiss clocks. The merchandise in all these stores is ordered, arranged, controlled. Everything smells new and unused, which is how *I* feel here, the way I wish I could always be.

□ □ □

One day in fifth grade I sit with my legs apart, showing my underpants. This act is willful, compulsive. I feel as if I *have* to do it, even as I know I don't want to do it. I feel as if I have to show someone—anyone—what I know how to do, even as I don't want to be noticed. In front of the class Miss DuVall tells me young ladies should never sit like that. I lower my eyes and don't want to return to school.

Besides, I don't quite understand school. We are given books to read, lessons to memorize, and while I vaguely understand that I am supposed to read the books and learn the lessons, I do not believe they are important. How can this knowledge help me? How can teachers teach me anything? Doesn't my father teach me all I need to know? Doesn't he always tell me so?

Why, then, do I lack words for what I know? At school we are taught French, but *still*, even in this language, I learn no words for what I know, for what I am taught at night. So if words don't exist, if definitions don't exist, if signs and symbols don't exist, then maybe people and actions don't exist either. None of us exists. Night doesn't exist. Bodies don't exist. I don't exist, for surely I know no language that might prove otherwise.

What is the definition of "father," "mother," "sister," "daughter," "soul," "family," "love"? Do I ever learn? Maybe all the definitions I learn are wrong.

I do learn, however, one of the most important lessons of my life: Contradictions never startle or surprise me. I am capable of living with irreconcilable contradictions.

□ □ □

I am a Brownie for one day, attend only one meeting, then refuse to return. Immediately I notice the badges the girls have sewn on their uniforms, badges proclaiming skills at which they excel, goals accomplished. I know the skills at which I excel. Even lacking words, I believe these are my only skills. But the badges worn by these girls don't portray beds, sheets, bodies. Does this mean my skills are useless? How do I know, though, lacking words, symbols, definitions, that no girl wears these badges because no badges are even designed that portray beds, sheets, bodies? All I know is that I can't return for the next Scout meeting. I couldn't bear to be the only Brownie with no badge sewn on her brown uniform.

□ □ □

One day at school we are served corn fritters for lunch. I know I cannot eat them. I know the moist, chunky pieces of corn embedded in a soggy white mass will make me sick. I stare at the plate, at the two fritters I am required to eat. Just from the smell my throat feels cold, my forehead sweaty. The headmistress says if I don't eat both of them I will be taken to the bathroom and punished. I am afraid of her, afraid of her bony fingers. I imagine them punishing me, imagine them scrubbing my mouth with soap. Billy whispers he'll eat mine if I slide them onto his plate, but the headmistress doesn't take her eyes off me. I hold my breath and slowly begin to eat. I take tiny bites, drinking milk between bites to wash away the taste. I am determined not to be sick at school—not in front of everyone. The milk is gone long before the fritters, and as the others file back to class I am left alone on the veranda with the headmistress and my fritters. My sister passes and refuses to look at me; I embarrass her. I know I do and would eat them for her sake alone if I could. It takes the rest of the afternoon—through French and math and recess—before I eat the last bite of fritter.

The school bus drives us down the mountain. Today I don't stay in town but climb the 99 Steps up to Blackbeard's Hill, up the hill to our house, to my bedroom. In the cool, silent house I lie on my bed, my skin sweating, my stomach freezing, waiting to throw up. I throw up for hours, on and off, unable to stop. My mother brings me ginger ale and presses damp washcloths to my forehead. I vomit every kernel of corn into the bucket she has placed on the floor next to my bed. I must get rid of it all. My mother disdains fried food and calls the headmistress in a rage: I am never to be forced to eat corn fritters again. But her rage is deeper: Our family is insular. No one from the outside world is allowed to interfere. It is she, she and my father only, who control what enters my body.

It is late at night before I finish being sick. I had fallen asleep and when I awake my father is sitting next to me. Through the windows the breeze feels cool and fresh. Fronds of coconut palms rustle. In the distance, a goat is bleating. When I move and my father realizes I am awake, he wipes my face with a wet cloth. This is all. He wipes my face and brushes hair from my forehead. I whisper to him I was sick. Gently, he squeezes my hand, then holds the glass of ginger ale to my lips. Slowly, I sip it. I want him to stay here, holding the glass, wiping my face. He has placed a small copper bell next to my bed and tells me to ring it if I wake up sick. He tucks the mosquito net under the mattress and I watch him leave. I want to say to him: *Stop, Daddy. Come back.* But I say nothing. He might ask why, and I'd have no answer. I will have to wait for years, until I am an adult, before I know what I would have said to him if I'd called him back. I would have said: *This is all it takes, this is all I want, this is how easy it is to be a father.*

□ □ □

Summers, we spend in the States. My mother takes my sister and me to New York City to visit her sister, my Aunt Patsy, and Uncle Evan. My father will join us later. I am particularly fond of my Uncle Evan and call him Esey. They have no children, and he spends hours playing with me. For a living, Esey writes jokes and books about jokes. He makes up word games and teaches me to play. His office is in their small apartment and the room is crammed, floor to ceiling, with bookshelves. I lie on the cranberry-colored carpet and gaze up at the green, brown, tan, black spines of the books. I love the way the room smells of old dusty paper and ink. The solidity of the books, the thousands and thousands of well-ordered words creating sentences, creating paragraphs, imparting information and knowledge, is reassuring, even though I don't yet have the desire to read the books, don't believe I would understand them. For now, I simply love being in the company of these books because Esey loves them.

Uncle Esey lets me distract him from his work when I am bored. I poke through cubbyholes of his rolltop desk, which is stuffed with notecards, bottles of ink, boxes of paper clips, rubber bands. I sit on his lap and peck at the keys on his black typewriter. He tells me funny stories. He has a soft smile and gentle hands, and I follow him around the apartment and go out with him to run errands. He takes me to the Museum of Natural History and spends hours with me when I discover the ancient Egyptian exhibits—the jewelry, the pottery, the artifacts. I am mesmerized by the display. I imagine her, *my* Egyptian princess, wearing silver and gold and smelling of the mysterious green water of the Nile.

Patsy and Esey take us to my first Chinese restaurant. My favorite part is the fortune cookie and Esey gives me his. I'm amazed that one's fortune can arrive serendipitously in a cookie. I save my slips of white paper as proof of a bright future. I believe in this, in the future, more than the present, certainly more than the past.

At dusk I stand at the window in their living room and watch lights bloom across Manhattan. We are high in a skyscraper, and I think of the mountains at home, standing on the terrace of the V. I. Hotel and gazing down at Charlotte Amalie. The island seems unreal and far away. I try to imagine my father alone up at the hotel while we, his three little girls, as he still calls us, are away from him. I wonder if he misses us. I know he does. He has to. He must. Before I left he whispered to me how much he would miss me, me, his most special, precious little girl. But maybe he's not alone at the hotel, I think. He hates to be alone. I feel slightly scared when I think of him dancing with another precious little girl.

I lie on the leather couch. Light from the rest of the apartment filters into the living room. From Esey's study comes the sound of typing. My sister is in the bedroom reading. She loves to read, to be alone, and I know better than to ask her to play with me. In the kitchen my mother talks to my aunt. Earlier in the day I had discovered a toy, a Hawaiian dancing girl, stuffed into a drawer in a bureau. It is about three inches high. The Hawaiian girl, made of rubber, wears a grass skirt, but her breasts are bare. She stands on a wood base and by turning a small lever her hips and breasts gyrate. I am entranced by this motion. I know my daddy must have bought this present for my uncle, for he is the one who traveled to Hawaii.

My father arrives in New York to take us to Monhegan Island in Maine. On his first night in the city he holds me on his lap while telling us all the news of St. Thomas. He is stroking my knee, and suddenly I am filled with dread when I think of the trip to Maine. I thought I had missed him, had been waiting to see him, but now I want to stay here with my Uncle Esey. Later I take the Hawaiian doll to bed with me, hiding it under the sheet. My father turns off the light after he kisses my sister and me good-night. His bay rum aftershave smells too foreign here in the city. It reminds me of there, back there in my four-poster mahogany bed in our house next to Blackbeard's Castle.

After my father leaves the room, I see her again, the Egyptian princess. It's night. She's running across the sands of the desert. An orange slice of a moon dazzles the water of the Nile and reflects on the gold and silver bangly bracelets encircling her arms and her wrists. Reeds slash at her ankles as she runs faster, fleeing an angry pharaoh. She hides in the shadow of the Sphinx, waiting for an Egyptian prince to save her. But the prince doesn't come. I can't sleep. I still hold the Hawaiian dancer, but she's no longer Hawaiian. She's the Egyptian princess. I don't understand why I grip her so tightly, my thumb against her throat. Nor do I understand why I must bite off one of her nipples.

□ □ □

By the time we reach Monhegan Island my father is in a rage. Nothing has gone right on the trip: the food, the car, the maps, the directions, the roads, the ferry ride, his children, his wife—all are wrong. My mother, sister, and I are sullen. So even though the white wood hotel is lovely, the island is lovely, no one wants to be here. We all want to be back home where we are more comfortable in our own small private furies. As we unpack, my mother makes a final stab at a vacation and suggests we all change immediately and head to the beach. But this beach is not like the Caribbean. The water is frigid, the shoreline rocky. My mother will not enter this water and sits on a rock to sun herself. My sister wanders off down the shore. My father marches into the ocean. Even though water is scary to me, I follow. I must. I know he wants someone to be with him, and I must be the one.

The cold water stuns me, but I pretend to love it, knowing this will please my father. My mother calls to me to come out—that I will catch pneumonia or polio. My father tells her to leave me alone, the water is fine. She persists. He screams at her to shut up, shut up, to leave me, leave him alone, if she doesn't stop bothering us, he'll . . .

I sink below the surface of the water. Their voices fade. All I hear is the deep throb of the ocean, connecting me to all oceans . . . and if I loosened my moorings I would be able to float back to the Caribbean, float to New York City to see my Uncle Esey, float . . .

In this murky water I see nothing. The sodden cold weighs me deeper and deeper. I close my eyes and expel my breath in a slow rush of bubbles. It is here, now, I lose my fear of water. It is here I discover its soothing lap, lap against my skin, rocking me. In this body-numbing water I can let go and float to a deep basin of the sea. My seaweed hair will drift about my shoulders. My skin turns to phosphorescence. My fingernails are delicate pink shells. My teeth are pearls. And I will dwell forever beneath a warm blanket of sand on the ocean floor.

But then I feel his hands on me, those hands, on my arms, yanking me. When I surface, all I hear are tattered remnants of words from my mother. "There, now, you satisfied—" By the time I open my eyes she has turned from us and is walking back to the cabin.

I shiver so much my legs feel wayward and useless. My father carries me from the water and arranges towels on the rocks, placing me on them. He rubs my arms and legs to warm me. Heat from the rock feels as if it radiates my skin, seeping along my spine to the backs of my limbs. At first this feels good. As he breathes deeply, though, I begin to feel as if I'm back under water—this time fighting for air. He pulls my hand under the leg of his bathing suit, but my numb hand has trouble gripping him there. I feel his tension: We're outside, hurry up and do this. If I don't do this correctly and quickly he will be angry. I try to concentrate. I must remember what he has taught me, *how* he has taught me to do this.

Yes, you Dina, you weren't in the water, you're not shivering, you can do this.

But her small hand, too, at this angle, has trouble. We, Dina and I, are lying on the rock and we can't turn. Her elbow is rigid against stone, but Dina, *you want to do this for him. You want this as much as he does.* She rubs him as hard as she can, but it's not hard enough. Perhaps he's worried someone will see us. We've never done this outdoors before, and I—my body is shamed. I feel stripped, exposed, naked. His tension grows. He hasn't seen me in several weeks, and if he doesn't get what he needs soon he will hurt us. He yanks aside the crotch of my suit but doesn't even bother to touch me, just stares, stares, stares at me. No, not at me, at it. He stares at it. *Yes, do this, Father, do this. If this will make it happen quicker, do it. Do whatever you want. Just do it.*

His voice is hoarse, whispering: "Open your mouth. We can't get any on the towel, open your mouth. Damnit. Hurry."

My mouth is frozen shut, but he's pulling up the leg of his suit farther as he moves up and over me. Someone will see, I think, someone will come walking along the rocks. My sister will return. My mother. I shut my own eyes, not wanting to witness this. It is Dina, Dina is finally able to open her mouth, and he shoves it against the roof of her mouth just as he ejaculates. But she can't swallow fast enough. Damn her, damn her. What's wrong with her? Maybe she's not used to sunlight either. Before, it's always been dark . . . Dina disappears, and now it is my throat. I can't swallow. I spit it out all over the towel. He lies back, and I think about lifting a rock and smashing him . . . No, I think, no. I must be perfect, and he will love me. I must clean up this mess I have made, do nothing to make him angry. I take the towel to the edge of the ocean and scrub it with sand. I scoop water into my mouth and swallow it, but still I taste it, that taste, and I put a handful of sand in my mouth and scrub it across my teeth and my tongue with a finger.

It is then I see my mother. My legs buckle and I sit flat on the sand. She's walking toward me over the rocks, and I don't know whether she saw us or not. My body feels as if she did see—it is weak with shame—and I believe that even from this distance she can smell that stuff in my mouth. I look down at my body. My father has not properly arranged the crotch of my suit, but my arms are unable to move in order to fix it. I am without will. And as I sit here, I think I see myself floating away, rising up from the shoreline, as if the ocean opened its mouth in a curl of a wave and released me in a spindrift. I float higher and higher, so by the time my mother reaches the spot where my body once was, I know it is not me she touches. It is not my mouth her fingers probe as she scoops out sand. It is not my ears threatened with her words. It is not my arm her fingernails puncture as she yanks me back to the cabin, passing my sleeping father without a word or a glance. Again, it is not my ears that hear her say I have sand in my crotch; if it's not properly cleaned, it will become infected. I am in a bathtub of icy water—icy, she says, to kill any germs that might cause infection. She separates my legs and washes the sand away with her hand. *Yes, do this, Mother,* I think. *Wash it away.* My mother will make me better. She is calmer now. The bottom of the tub is gritty with sand, but as soon as she pulls the plug it will disappear forever. Everything will be fine, she tells me. We'll just get you cleaned up. We'll wash the sand from your hair. You have such pretty hair.

By the time I am clean and dry and dressed, my father has returned to the cabin. He, too, is now calm. Yes, my mother is right: Everything will be better now. I know this. He just needed to do that. Then he is calm and better. We're all better. He sits in a chair reading the *New York Times* and barely glances at us as we enter.

I leave the cabin and go to the lobby of the hotel. Through a picture window overlooking the ocean, I see my sister far down the beach jumping from rock to rock. If she tripped and fell . . . I want her to, but not because I hate her. I want her to fall so I can rush out and save her. She would be indebted to me forever. She would love me forever, love me more than she loves to be alone. Except my sister will never trip. Insistently, her ramrod body will refuse ever to stumble, ever to waver, ever to fall. So why, then, do I feel so sad watching her?

I wander into the dining room where college kids on vacation set tables for dinner. I watch a girl with shiny blonde hair pour water from a pitcher into a glass. Her skin looks healthy and scrubbed. She wears lipstick the color of pink pop-it beads, and she smiles at me with white-white teeth as she wanders over. I want her to like me. I want to be her friend. She says her name is Trixie, and immediately I love the solid sound of her name, the way her tongue ticks the roof of her mouth when it hits the hard "x" and "t." Solid, yes, and I wish I had a solid name, not the too-soft, too-weak whisper of a fading vowel. To myself, I say her name over and over and smile back. She asks if I'm hungry, and when I nod she brings me a piece of chocolate cake. When I finish, she brings me another. I want her to invite me to go with her to college.

That night at dinner she is our waitress. What luck, I think, as I see her bring us menus. But now I'm worried my father won't like the food, that he'll raise his voice at Trixie, that he will send food back to the kitchen. I'm so scared I can't eat much dinner. Besides, I'm full of chocolate cake. All I eat are a couple of rolls and another piece of cake. But my father likes the food. He also likes Trixie. He jokes with her, asks where she goes to college, asks if she has boyfriends. "You must have loads of boyfriends," he says, smiling. When she pours him a cup of coffee he pats her hip, and the three of us, his three little girls, sit hunched inside ourselves, silent.

For two weeks I only eat cake and rolls. Trixie feeds me cake between meals as if she knows I'm hollow and she will be the one to fill me. So I eat and eat and eat. The more cake I eat, the more ravenous I become, and could eat even more cake than offered but am too shy to ask. I eat until I am drunk on sugar. Later, all I can do is sit on the rocks or sleep. I don't go for walks. I can't go swimming—I am too bloated. Too dizzy. Too stuffed. When I awake I feel hungover and must return to Trixie to feed me more and more cake, until no longer do I remember what my father and I did together on the beach.

I get sick. My skin and my eyes yellow. For days I lie in bed, finally completely stuffed and unable to eat one more bite of cake. I want my mother to comfort me, sit beside me, tell me she loves me. She doesn't. She can't. She doesn't seem to know how to love me, but of course who could possibly love this bloated yellow body? Trixie visits, but just seeing her I think of sugar and I wait for her to leave. When my father talks to her he stands close to her and puts his hand on her arm when he smiles. She tells my parents a newly arrived hotel guest is a doctor. My mother asks him if he will see me. The doctor gives me enemas, but this strange man touching my body doesn't scare me. My body no longer feels shame. Finally, I feel nothing.

□ □ □

From Maine we stop in New York for a few days to see my aunt and uncle before returning to the West Indies. It is late September. The Antilles School will start soon. In this early fall, the leaves in Central Park are red and yellow. I remember the fall in second grade, in Maryland, when I couldn't attend school and try to think back to that time, try to remember why I stayed home, but that seems like another little girl afraid of school, another little girl afraid to leave her mother.

□ □ □

I'm not yet old enough to attend the dance at the Grand Hotel for the young Danish sailors who sail to port aboard the *Danmark*, but I want to meet a sailor. I must go. Earlier in the day my friends and I watched the square-rigged training ship glide around the point by Hassel Island. The bow gently plowed and furrowed the blue water. Wind puffed the rows of square-rigged sails. As the ship neared port I saw the blurred outlines of sailors swabbing the deck, getting ready for the islanders who would come aboard to visit. The *Danmark* dropped anchor next to the yellow bauxite on the pier, the silver flecks in the bauxite reflecting tiny wands of sunlight till it shimmered. I must meet a sailor. I want to dance with one.

Without letup I beg my mother. She keeps saying no. I will leave early, I say. She can fetch me any time she wants, but I must go. "I have to go," I say. "I'm going."

Finally she relents. My father puts on his linen jacket and says he has to work late. Since the bank is only a block from the Grand Hotel, he says, he'll pick me up afterwards.

My mother helps me dress in my red and black dress with tiny black buttons and black patent-leather shoes. I slip a long strand of white pop-it beads around my neck. I ask her to braid my ponytail, and she does. When I am ready, I walk carefully down the 99 Steps, scared I'll scuff a shoe, rip a hem, mess my hair. I have to be perfect. I have to be asked to dance, for this will make me perfect.

At first, though, I don't think about dancing, because all I can see is the dance itself. *It* is perfect, exactly the way it should be. The girls' dresses look like butterfly wings fluttering across the dance floor. The sailors' uniforms are as white as the foam on the waves at Magens Bay, with the word *Danmark* embroidered in gold on black cap-bands. Their unfamiliar accents circle the whorls of my ears. I feel as if they've traveled the world, yes, and brought all the world with them, here to this dance, here to me.

From across the room I notice a sailor watching me. Most of the sailors are blonde, but this one isn't. His black hair, I know, will smell like the mysterious depths of the sea. I glance away from him, down at the floor. I step back. For a moment I remember the way Billy smells in the forest: of fresh lime trees and the sun. The sailor is different. I know this. And then I understand that if he is different, I must be, too. I am not like these other girls. So as much as I want him to ask me to dance, as much as I want to dance, I don't want him to know me, know I am not like these other girls, in their soft pastel dresses. I am in red and black. I should not have braided my ponytail. I should not have worn this long strand of plastic pearls. I am . . . I am another kind of girl, and I believe he must know it.

He walks toward me. I hold my breath. He doesn't ask me to dance, but he takes my hand. Even though he doesn't hold me tight, still, with his hand pressed to my back, I feel stifled and trapped. My chin brushes his starched uniform and feels as if it's been burned. Yet if he leads me from the dance, if he leads me to his ship, I will have to follow. I will go with him, even though if he touches my body my father will know.

I see now I should not have come to the dance. No longer can I hear music. The girls' dresses, the sailors' uniforms, the dancing couples seem flat, muted. I am too far away to see. With the sway of his body the sailor edges me outside to the second-story veranda overlooking Emancipation Park and the harbor where the *Danmark* is anchored. Still we are dancing, but slower. He is dancing with Dina, and he must know it. From the moment he saw me he knew who I was: a girl who would dance outside with a stranger. He pauses by the rail and brushes a strand of hair from my forehead. *No, don't do this, stop.* But he can't hear the words. From his pocket he removes a white and blue silk handkerchief with an image of the *Danmark* on it. He gives it to me, a present, but I believe it is payment—I understand what is expected, what I am supposed to do in order to be able to keep it. Still, I take it. I want it. I smile at him. He bends to hold me again, and I must let him. I don't know how to stop. He is bending closer and closer—and maybe it's only to dance with me, but . . .

It is now, at this moment, I feel *him,* the other him, leaving the bank, my father, who knows now is the time he must come to get me. He is turning off the lights in the bank. He is locking the wrought-iron grill behind him. He is walking toward the car. He will be the one to save me—the only one capable of saving me. And as the sailor bends closer I believe I see, from the corner of my eye, headlights from my father's car beam up the street toward the Grand Hotel, searching for me. He knows I am calling to him, knows he must come for me. The only way I can stop dancing with the sailor is with the help of my father. I have promised my father that nothing would ever happen to my body, which is me.

I pull away from the sailor. Back away. Immediately he lets go, doesn't force me to stay. Instead he is smiling, asking if he has done something wrong. I shake my head and hold out the handkerchief, returning it. He says, no, keep it, it's for you, I want you to have it. I'm not sure I understand. I thought the present meant . . .

Maybe he only wants to dance. But I feel the headlights, closer. I turn and run.

Driving up the mountain with my father, I watch the harbor. The moon, or perhaps it is the bright headlights of my father's car, weaken the lights outlining the masts of the *Danmark*. The horizon from which the ship sailed is lost to the sky. Then the road winds around the mountain, and the harbor is no longer visible. My father holds my hand and squeezes it. He pulls me closer, trailing his fingers up my leg to the beginning of my thigh, there, and without hesitation I do what I've been taught, separate my legs, and he can't can't can't wait until we get home. His fingers touch my underpants and he must . . . He stops the car on the dark street. He pulls off my underpants and unzips his slacks. He edges me down on the seat, on my back, and leans over me. He is so close to me, he is all I can see, and that part of him that he wants me to love is hard against me, not yet in me but against me, pinning me to him, and I can't move. "Tell me you hated it," he says. "The dance."

"Yes, Daddy, I hated it."

He kisses me and touches my body. "You want to be with me."

"Yes, Daddy," I whisper.

And then he is pinning me deeper. The top of my head bangs the door handle as he does what he does when he has to be inside of me. I concentrate on that, on the top of my head hitting metal as he loves me loves me loves me almost more than either of us can manage. He does it, and as he does it the ship, the clipper ship from Denmark—I feel it sailing far away from me. But wait, I think. It has to wait: I realize I forgot to thank the sailor for the present. I have to thank him. But he is gone, and I scream, "Daddy, stop it"—and I mean the ship. I think I mean the ship, that I want him to stop the ship from sailing away, want him to bring the sailor back. But my father doesn't hear me. And he will never be able to stop it.

The next morning my mother comes in my bedroom and throws the silk handkerchief on my bed. I had dropped it in the car the night before. She asks who gave it to me. I tell her a sailor—just a sailor—I don't know his name. Did you dance with him much? she wants to know. "No, only just once," I say. Did he try to kiss you? she asks. "No, Mom, of course not," I say, laughing. Did he hold you? He must have kissed you. "No, Mom, no, no, no." I begin to scream—but no, it's a laugh. I laugh harder. "Nothing happened." She insists something did, I must have done something or he wouldn't have given me such a present. But all I can do is pound my fists on the bed and laugh.

□ □ □

At least once a week, when my mother is not watching, I steal a penny out of her wallet. Back in my room I retrieve my Chinese puzzle box that I keep hidden under my doll clothes. The box has a secret chamber that releases the lock. I spring it open. And each week I add another penny to my collection.

□ □ □

My mother is too sick to get out of bed. I hurry home from school every afternoon to sit with her while she listens to her radio, waiting for the news. I press cold washclothes on her forehead. I stroke her hand. Nothing I do helps her feel better. The doctor, she says, must be called. For days, every day, he comes to see her, even though every day she worsens—with an illness given no name or explanation. Only when the doctor is examining her, are her eyes brighter, bluer. On his way out the door, I hear her thin voice urging him back tomorrow.

My father views illness as an unwelcome intrusion into his need for order and control, so he spends less time at home, eating most of his meals at the hotels. In the emergency my sister spends more time at home, baking chocolate cakes for our breakfasts and cream puffs, in the shape of swans, for our dinners. She arranges the swans on a mirror while I set the table, using our best linen, china, and silver. I light candles and we sit across from each other, just the two of us. Slowly, we pluck swans off the mirror. Slowly, we disassemble each one. With small, delicate bites we munch wings, necks, heads, tails, before slowly licking cream from the bodies. When the mirror reflects no more swans, my sister and I gaze at each other, stuffed and satisfied by this quiet dinner, by this quiet house, by this quiet night. I drift asleep, dizzy on sugar. I wake up dizzy, go to school dizzy, after eating a slab of chocolate cake, craving this dizziness, this distraction, which helps me to forget everything else.

□ □ □

The movie *Limelight*, with Charlie Chaplin, plays at the cinema. It is the story of a young ballerina who suffers hysterical paralysis and tries to commit suicide. An older man, Chaplin, saves her, then continues to nurture her, love her, cure her. After the movie my weeping is uncontrollable—*I* am. I am inconsolable. This man Charlie Chaplin must be my savior, even though it is far from possible for me to voice from what it is I need to be saved. *This*, this older man, is the man who must be my father, my lover, my . . . I barely know what I want or need from him, but the need is boundless. I am restless. Anxious. I can't eat. I'm unable to sleep. For days I can't leave the house.

Even when I finally go outside again and lie in a field shaded by tamarind trees, he is with me. He never leaves. I hear him in the rattle of pods on the trees. I feel him in the grass beneath my legs, hear him as spiders strum their silky webs. I feel safe here, with him in this field. He will keep me safe—my savior.

□ □ □

One evening while my mother is still sick and my father is out Maria calls to tell me she is running away from home. She wants me to meet her in Emancipation Park and bring her food. I gather the remains of a chocolate cake, a loaf of bread, and a couple of 7-Ups before hurrying down the mountain. She waits for me on a wrought-iron bench. Light from the Grand Hotel spills across the park, and immediately I see that her nose is bloody and beginning to swell. I know her father has hit her. She has been crying—she's not now, but her lashes are wet. I tell her the first thing we must do is clean off her nose, and I lead her across the park to the harbor.

She's not feeling well and lies on the dock. I'd wrapped the cake in a dish towel, which I remove and dip into the water to clean her. When I dab at her nose she winces from the pressure. We need help. We need ice to stop the swelling, but there's no place downtown to get it where I won't be questioned. Billy is the only person I can think of who might help us, but I'd have to go to the Grand or the Hotel 1829 to use a phone and, again, I would be questioned.

Maria says she's going to be sick. Quickly, I try to open the 7-Up for her but realize I've forgotten an opener. I feel terrible, angry at myself for being so stupid. She rolls onto her stomach and vomits into the harbor, careful not to make a mess. I tell her I have to get help—maybe the police or a doctor—that she can't run away with a bloody nose, and there's nowhere to run anyway. On an island, where would she go?

She wants to stow away on an ocean liner, she says. Sometimes, she says, she sits in her bedroom window for hours staring at the horizon, imagining herself crossing it, crossing to the other side. "I hate it here," she says. "I don't know why we have to live here. I wish we could go back to San Juan."

But I don't see how she can leave. Tonight no cruise ships are in port. Except for lights from the Grand and the faint sound of music from its bar, the downtown is deserted.

"What'd you do?" I say, motioning toward her nose.

"My daddy goes through my stuff and found this math test. He was mad I only got a *B*. And—I don't know—I guess I got mad back at him. I shouldn't have done that."

"Is he still mad?"

She shrugs. "I mean he just slapped me—and I kind of tripped and fell. You know how clumsy I am."

I know her father is still mad. And I know she shouldn't return home until morning. So I ask her if she has any money, thinking we can take a taxi to the hotel, where Billy might be able to sneak her into one of the cabanas.

But Maria has no money. So I say I'll have to risk going to the Grand to call Billy, see if he'll come down the mountain and get us. After all, we can't stay on the dock all night.

She shrugs okay, that I can call Billy.

I cross the park to the Grand, but run into my father. He is under the canopy in front of the hotel saying good-night to a man and a woman who work for him. As I approach, the two move off toward Government Hill, and my father puts his hand on my arm. But we have nothing to say. We stare at each other speechless, almost shyly, it seems, or embarrassed. Because of who we are to each other? What can he say to this girl who's his daughter, but isn't—this girl who's a stranger? He has no idea who I am or what I might do, or be, when I'm away from him. So at first he doesn't even know how to ask why I'm here, perhaps suspecting I've met Billy or one of the boys from school. I don't want to tell him about Maria, but—my mind races—the truth or a lie?—which would be safer? With his hand on my arm, I feel immobilized. He will not let go until I tell him something; I know this. Maria is sick, I finally say.

I lead him to the harbor where he kneels beside her. While one hand holds her chin, he gently examines her nose with the other. I see her neck strain from his touch, but only barely. I know she won't tell him to stop either. I look away from them—see only night. At night the horizon is lost to opaque space. I know Maria will never be able to reach it, not even during the day when she can see it. The island is too still. Banana boats gently knock against the dock, but this is the only sound.

He asks who did this to her. She shakes her head. She won't say. "One of the islanders," he guesses, even though he sees himself as their champion, the one to come here to "save" them from poverty. "Which one? I'll have him arrested."

Maria shakes her head harder. "No," she says, "nothing like that."

"Tell me," he says. "I'll take care of this. It was one of the boys from school?"

"No," I say, my voice angry. "It was her father. That's who did this."

His look of disbelief is sincere, I know this. He rocks back on his heels before standing. "Her father would never do this," he says. There's not a shred of irony on his face or in his voice, and once again I know that I have no idea who this man is. It is this that scares me, at the moment, more than anything. "I know him."

"Why not?" I say. "Fathers—"

He whirls toward me so fast I think he might hit me. "What?" he says. "Tell me."

But my throat is stuffed with the hard, cold sound of his voice and I look away from him, saying nothing.

"I know you girls. You got into some trouble with boys and you're lying. Tell me."

He wants a name. He wants a lie. If I could have thought of a lie, a lie without implicating others, I would tell it, just to get this over with. But short of saying I'd bloodied Maria's nose myself which, if I thought he'd believe, I would have, I think of nothing.

"Anyway, what difference does it make what happened?" I say. "She needs a doctor."

"That will be up to her parents. It's not our place. Of course, they'll call the doctor."

He says he'll take her home. She doesn't object. She, as well as I, knows the futility.

Maria and I silently wait at the dock while my father brings the car around. She lies in the back seat, I sit in front, and we drive deserted streets past Market Square, past French Town. At Maria's house all the lights are off. No one has waited up for her; no one has gone looking. I know there will be no call to a doctor, but I say nothing, no more suggestions, abandoning her, yes, I know this. As soon as she is out of the car, my father drives off, not waiting to see whether she makes it safely inside. But of course that's where the danger is, inside. So why wait?

My father is angry—I know this, too. Angry because he believes I've lied? Or is his anger darker? Does he think I've just judged him, not Maria's father? But perhaps he doesn't think about this. Perhaps he doesn't think about himself and me at all. Perhaps he's more truly lost even than I.

But my own rage is now emerging—although I don't understand it as rage. Rather, it feels like suffocation. I can barely breathe. I can't swallow. As the car curves up the mountain, I am silenced by the strength of this feeling. We both are silenced. But I can feel my father's hands grip the steering wheel, feel the force of his hand shifting gears, hear the grating of metal as the engine strains against the incline all the way to our house.

Tonight he doesn't wait for me to go to bed first, doesn't pretend he comes to my bedroom simply to say good-night. Tonight I will be punished for what I have done. There is rage in his hands as he yanks off my shirt, rage in his heart as he yanks off my shorts. He will see no contradiction. No inconsistency. Soon, neither will I. This makes perfect sense to him. Even in his rage he calls this love and believes this, *this*, and only this will absorb and blunt the rage exploding out the tops of our skulls. And he is right. In terror my rage peaks, and my rage, now mine, knifes away into Dina, lovingly transmogrified into desire, and she, oh how she craves him. His hand grips her ponytail, slamming her head up and down, her mouth around his penis. And I . . . I float far away from Dina and am blessedly safe, safe with my daddy who loves me.

It is morning. Early. No one is yet awake, but my father is still in bed with me. I am naked; we are both naked. Perhaps because my mother is sick, this is the first time he stays the night. It is like the time at Monhegan Island when we were outside on the beach. Again I feel too exposed, too shy. Sun terrifies me. All night I thought I heard the spinneret of a spider weaving a marquisette net to hide us. But it is too flimsy. The harsh sun will melt it. I have no will and nowhere to hide. As my father wakes he pulls me toward him. And when he enters me I feel as if he seeps through every vein beneath my skin.

□ □ □

After school I climb Government Hill that leads to the 99 Steps and Blackbeard's Hill and Castle. I zigzag steep slopes, easier than walking straight up. Magenta bougainvillea vines droop over whitewashed stucco fences with wrought-iron gates. I press my palms flat against the whitewash, then lean against the wall to color my skin and clothes chalk-white, pretending I am invisible, that my only existence is the imprint of my body in the whitewashed wall.

Finally, by summer, I no longer believe in my existence and believe I am disappearing, deep inside sleep. In my whitened image I am fading, am almost asleep. My diminished, whitewashed body is will-less, unable to withstand the physical force of sleep that seems to drift toward me like the trade winds, slowly, as if gathering velocity from across the sea. I am powerless. I want to be powerless. I welcome sleep, its massive, numbing presence flowing toward me from the horizon. I watch it daily, motionless at one end of its gray, engulfing path. Every day I am more drowsy and soon all I can do is lie in my bed and wait.

When it arrives I feel as if it is lifting me, transporting me on wind currents until I am no longer here. Voices grow hazy. Faces and objects blur. Does someone call, searching for me? No longer do I recognize the sound of my name. In this sheer strength of sleep—as profound as a language of utter silence—all other movement, all other sound, all whispers of dark Caribbean nights are deflected. I am unable to hear. I am carried too far away from my mahogany bed even to see my sleeping body veiled in marquisette netting.

Yet those moments when I skim the surface of sleep I feel our maid, Sylvanita, dampen my arms and face and neck with a cool balm scented with khuskhus. It doesn't wake me. The scent only seems to deepen with sleep.

After three months I awake. I awake slowly, sluggishly, not refreshed from sleep, still groggy, struggling to breathe. I stand outside on the terrace, stunned by sunlight. It sears the rims of my eyes. I gaze at the fathomless, indecipherable sea: It is still here. The yellow-orange sun still blisters the Caribbean sky. Right before sunset, limestone dust seems to converge high in the air, blocking cool trade winds for just that moment. Tiny particles burn the sky red with heat.

□ □ □

All year I wait for Carnival, when the island itself seems decorated with masks and feathers and flowers. The park is crisscrossed with colored lights, while Carnival booths are adorned with crepe and palm fronds. I watch the dancers, hear the rush and rustle of madras skirts, the pong of steel-drum bands. I pass booths selling coconut balls, fried plantains, orange wine, stewed cashews, sugar cake. I buy a guava ice and stand under a lignum vitae tree licking it, watching the moko-jumbis, invisible spirits who walk on stilts. They wear mirrored costumes so no one can see them. When you look at them you see yourself. I imagine my own body camouflaged with tiny glass mirrors.

After I finish the ice I cross the park to a beautiful booth draped in silver scarves and gold lights. An old woman, her hair wrapped in a head tie, leans against the counter next to a hurricane lantern. The sign tacked to the booth reads: CUP OF SNAKE WEED TEA/.25—GLASS OF CLAIRIN/.75.

I place four quarters on the counter. "Can I have some?" I ask. I've never heard of the drinks, but I like the sound of the names.

She takes only one quarter, telling me I'm too young for clairin but she'll give me a cup of the tea.

From a pitcher she pours a dark liquid into a tiny china cup. Drinking it, I seem to taste tree roots after a tropical storm. At first the taste is mild, but at the bottom of the cup is a thick, rich residue. And I wonder if this is a black magic potion. I think it must be, and I wonder if I will now have secret powers.

Returning the cup to her I smile, thanking her.

"You like it?" she says.

"Yes."

She nods and tells me I have a pretty smile.

My fingers rush to my lips as if to feel this smile. This concrete information seems overwhelmingly important. *A pretty smile.* On my own face. Now, I don't so much want to be a moko-jumbi as I want to be able to *look* at a moko-jumbi, at his mirrors, in order to see this smile, one I myself never noticed.

Slowly I move past thinning crowds. This last night of Carnival, booths are being dismantled, decorations folded for next year, and I realize I don't want Carnival to end. I want to live here in this Carnival with moko-jumbis and with steel-drum bands. I want to live with the woman and her snake weed tea. If she feeds me weed tea every morning I will smile. But Carnival is over. I fear I'll never see this woman again. She has given me a special tea that has given me a special, secret power—my special smile. Is she the only one who can see my true-true smile?

Why does my father see something, someone different? I have a special smile that my own daddy can't see, even when he is very close to me.

☐ ☐ ☐

My mother's illness continues, and my father finally arranges for her to see a doctor in New York City. She will love this, I know; she will love to be able to see a new doctor, let a new doctor see her. My parents will stay in my Aunt Patsy and Uncle Esey's apartment while they come to the island to care for my sister and me. But I am told of these arrivals and departures only the night before. Terror that my mother will never return becomes rage, becomes a tantrum. What I don't know is that this is the last tantrum I will ever have. By the time my parents return, I will have outgrown them. But I must have this last one, for I believe if I scream loudly enough my mother will hear me and won't leave me. I believe if I fling myself against the bureau and cut my forehead, this will keep her home.

Nothing will keep her home.

After my parents are gone, I am quiet. The house is quiet, recovering from my kicks and punches. I lie on the couch and watch a shaft of sun sprinkle my sister's canary in light. On the table beside the cage are my mother's watercolor paints and unfinished paintings. They are very good. They are almost her life. But they aren't enough for her life. Neither am I. Or my sister. Or my father. We are not enough to hold her attention. It is her illness she nurtures, that she watches develop and grow.

Without my parents my own life feels diminished, even though Esey tries to cheer me. He reads to me and tells me stories. He plays marbles with me, listens to my make-believe games. The marbles are pirates saving maidens in distress. The pirates rescue me and sail me to New York City. Esey and I play with my dolls, my five Annettes, dressing them in hats, plastic shoes, frilly dresses. We pack their tiny cardboard suitcases for their trip to New York to visit my parents—which is where *I* want to be. So even my Uncle Esey can't truly cheer me as I wait for my parents. Every day I write letters to tell them I miss them.

At night, Esey tucks me in my bed and tells me a story. I'm afraid to let him leave me, and I make him promise to stay in my room until he's positive I'm sleeping, protecting me from spirits that hide in folds of mosquito nets, that hide behind shadows in the darkest corner of the room.

But Esey isn't strong enough to protect me from these spirits. Esey can't hear the danger in the flap of bird wings that shatters the quiet of night. Only my own father truly knows how to watch over me, knows where my body is and how to protect it . . .

It is late afternoon when I walk to town for the mail to see if there are letters from my mother and father. At the bank, where our mail is delivered, I stop to talk to the people who work for my father. There *is* a letter from my parents, but I will wait to read it, postpone the excitement until I am home. By waiting, I will imagine all the wonderful things the letter will say: how they miss me and love me and will be home soon. When I leave the bank I run into Patti, who invites me to Katz's for a Coke—her treat. Then we pause to admire the display of lipsticks on the counter.

By the time I head back up the mountain it is dusk, and under the trees, almost night. Partway up is a low cement wall fencing an overgrown park. Because I feel bouyant, happy with the letter, which I stick in the elastic waistband of my shorts, I jump up on the ledge and do a few ballet steps, balancing, knowing I can't fall. My arms are outstretched, bent at the elbows, as I bend and weave.

I do not see the man, nor do I hear him. A cool hand, high up my thigh, stops me. A friendly voice offers assistance: I might fall; he will catch me. His arm has a blue tattoo. A sailor. At first I think to smile my special weed tea smile. But, no, he would not see it. He is switchblade thin and unsmiling, and I stand rigid, staring into pale, frosty eyes.

His fingers are beneath my underpants now, and all I can think is that they're cold. I feel as if I have stood here forever, but it can't be—it's just that the island night is slowing toward sleep. I feel this warm sleep of the island at my back, pressing against me like a sultry wind. I am lifted from the ledge. I am carried into the underbrush. My shorts are pulled from my body. And the sailor, his lips against my ear, whispers harsh words unheard before that describe my body. He is angry—the rape is too smooth for him, too easy—this girl's body is not what it first seemed. No obstacle leads into her body, so she is a cuntcuntcunt. *Yes, sailor, you are the only one who knows my secret: You are not my first lover.*

He is gone. I pull on my underpants and shorts and walk home. My walk is different, though. I can feel it—the slow-slow movement of my legs. My knees are looser. My hips feel slightly broader. I am molting. With every step, pieces of Dina slough from my skin and slip to my feet. I step past them, leaving them, walking away from this childbody that now seems nothing but useless trouble. In the raw tissue remaining on my skin from where Dina has eroded, the first cells of Celeste form.

Back up the mountain, I push open the rusty gate to Blackbeard's Castle. I follow the overgrown path that leads to the round stone fortress and sit on the stoop. Through tree branches and bushes I see the lights from my house, but I am hidden. My aunt and uncle don't know where I am. No one knows where I am. The night is lit with a tropical moon, but even the moon can't see me.

No one can see me. For now someone else breathes inside my chest. I feel a small throb in my temple. I lean back and press my head hard against the metal door of the fortress to steady myself, a self that seems to be shifting, evolving, moving, flowing. My hands, loose in my lap, curl into fists.

It is Celeste's hands that are strong, hands that make fists. Silky blonde hair billows down my back. My own pale lips turn the color of garnet, as Celeste slowly usurps my childhood body . . . and I know that with one strong breath Celeste is the one who can banish danger. With one blow of her fist she can smash the metal door and take possession of the stone fortress. For she is stronger than pirates, stronger than sailors who prowl the island at night. Stronger than my uncle. Stronger than any father. Stronger than any weed tea or secret potion. She is the one who now protects me. When my father returns he will find her, find Celeste, a girl unafraid of night spirits. She is a cunt. She is a slut. Much bolder than Dina. Celeste will look all rapists straight in the eye and smile.

I stand up and head toward my house. I touch the waistband of my shorts. The letter, that I no longer need to read, has vanished.

□ □ □

My sister is in eighth grade. Now too old to attend the Antilles School, she leaves the island to attend a private school in the States. Although she spent little time at home, the house seems lonely without her. Always I waited for her to explode into the house, if only to change her clothes, before again exploding out. Her energy awed and overwhelmed me. The more she raced across the island, the more I felt immobilized, waiting for her to come back. Now, after she's gone, I search every desk and bureau drawer in her bedroom, believing I'll find a memento that will reveal my sister's heart. *Kiki, what are your secrets? Who do you become when you so easily slip away from our house?* In some unswept corner of her room I want to discover her secrets as if I can discover her, an essence of her—to steal, to know, to understand, to become.

I find nothing. No secrets. No clues. Her room is swept bare. The dresser drawers are empty. Her closet holds only a thin rattle of hangers.

□ □ □

At first my mother seems better after her return from New York, but she's still not well. While some days she paints for hours before returning to bed, other days the paints are untouched and the shutters in her room remain shut. Finally, she decides it is the island that causes her illness, and we must return to the States right away. Besides, she believes Kiki will be better off living with her family. So six months after my sister leaves, we prepare to follow. My father arranges for the bank, the West Indies Bank and Trust Company, to be sold to Chase Manhattan.

As much as I once wanted to leave the States and live in the tropics, I now, just as much, want to leave the tropics and live in a cold, cold climate. I want to wear cashmere sweaters. I want to watch swirling snowflakes and skid on ice. I have an unshakable confidence in new homes, new environments, new habitats, new beginnings. I am also excited about seeing my sister. Surely she has missed me and will be happy to see me, although her letters give no indication. Besides, I am tired of my island friends, or so I pretend. Most truly I am afraid to feel close to them. I later learn I will always be relieved to move, especially away from people and things I most care about.

Still, I spend long hours saying good-bye to my friends. I say good-bye to guinea grass, hibiscus flowers, coconut palms, royal poincianas. Flying away on Caribair from St. Thomas to Puerto Rico, I sit by the window and watch the Caribbean flash viridian, aquamarine, turquoise, amethyst: blue. I say good-bye to the Caribbean, to red flowers, to green volcanic mountains. I am sad, after all. I believe I see a small girl standing on the shoreline, waving. She waves to me. She beckons. Wait. She stands alone, the hem of her skirt, strands of her hair swirling in the wind. Sunlight pushes against her back, and she runs down the beach, following the shadow of the plane. The plane veers north. Soon she is left far, far behind. I press my nose to the window, but the beach is deserted. The island vanishes. I don't want to lose her. But I already have.

New Jersey Girl

Glen Rock, New Jersey: 1958–1964

Winter. St. Thomas's red, green, blue mute to white snow, brown trees, New Jersey asphalt. An opaque iron sky replaces crimson sunsets, usurps colors that stream from the red core of the sun. Our house has no porch, no veranda. All the windows are shut tight. Only one door leads to my blue bedroom, where I now sit on my bed, staring at foreign feet, huge and plodding in thick white socks and heavy saddle shoes. I can't wear my buffalo-hide sandals and hadn't realized I would miss them. The French madras jumpers are packed away. I wear a blue-green wool checked skirt and matching crew-neck sweater. My body feels weighted in clothes. My hair is in a tight ponytail, tugging my scalp. It's my first day of school. I am in seventh grade. And I dread it.

The red brick school is divided into junior and senior high. My sister turns one way, I the other. I pass rows of metal lockers, not even searching for mine, not wanting to abandon, not even unzipping, my brown suede jacket trimmed with white fur. I'm afraid I'll look wrong, afraid I am wrong, afraid my body, away from sunlight and sea, has a terrible odor. While I have no particular thoughts, at this moment, of last night, I have a vague sense that if

I unzip my jacket something no one is supposed to see will be visible.

I want to be invisible. I stare at the linoleum floor, awed by the number of students, by crowded halls, by slamming lockers, by the rush of scuffing feet. Kids brush past, saying nothing. I grip a piece of paper that tells me which homeroom to locate, but I can't find it and am afraid to ask. Worse, I must change rooms every hour, for every class. I'm confused by all the identical doors, the identical rooms. I want the large, open, quiet windows overlooking the Caribbean. I want the waves of Magens Bay lapping, the scent of ginger flowers, the mist of egrets winging toward the mangrove swamp at dusk. I want my old schoolroom. My seat will be empty. I want my seat back. I know if I take one more step along this corridor I will scream. But no, I would never scream. Rather, I simply want to disappear, wanting no one to witness my desolation.

Bells have rung. Everyone else is seated when I finally stand in front of the class and hand the piece of paper to the homeroom teacher. My gaze doesn't leave my saddle shoes. They look too new, and I wish I'd scuffed them outside on the pavement. The teacher introduces me, tells everyone I'm from St. Thomas, as if this is exciting news. I know no one in the classroom will agree. Here, everyone must be the same, look the same, be from the same place, to be accepted. Without being told, I *know* this. Mortified, I grip my notebook to my chest. There is silence in the room. No one shouts a hello. More than anything, they're probably bored. The teacher asks if I want to remove my jacket—haven't I found my locker yet? I might want to hang my jacket in my locker. I know I must appear a dimwit, as if I'm unable to understand the language. I know, I *know* I must remove my jacket or be further humiliated, but I'm holding the notebook. I'm afraid I'll drop it if I try to unzip the jacket. Besides, I don't want to remove it. I want to hide my body; my body doesn't want to be here. If it is safely tucked inside this jacket it can pretend it's not here; it is still on the beach in St. Thomas. I am paralyzed now, unable to move. And by not being more responsive to the teacher, I know I make her angry. She points to an empty desk toward the back of the room. I slink toward it.

By mistake I'm assigned to an advanced science class. Again I awkwardly stand in front of the room as the teacher questions my credentials, adding that if I think I can handle the advanced class he'll be pleased to try. No. I shake my head, no, still unable to speak. Can't the teacher see by looking at me I would fail an advanced class? Can't he see I'll fail even the regular class, possibly fail everything? So far today I have taken no notes. In fact I feel that I *don't* understand the language. I am too confused by all the students in all the desks, confused by shuffling feet and paper, by hot, steamy classrooms.

As I turn to leave the science room, she enters: Jane. Even though I don't of course truly know her name now, surely I must guess her name simply by her presence. For it is a New Jersey name, just as she is a New Jersey girl. Her name is clean and simple, confident in the impact of its unconfusing syllable, a name with the feel of a firm handshake. I want Jane, this blonde-haired girl named Jane, for my friend forever, for life. For the first time all day I smile. She stares straight through me as if I am glass. And my body—yes, the feeling is in my body—feels as dark and as grim as a fever.

Right before lunch I find my locker, finally ready to relinquish my jacket. I've never opened a combination lock and am struggling, not able to understand how it works. My notebook, books, and jacket are by my feet—I've piled them almost on top of my shoes because I'm afraid to take up too much space in the crowded corridor.

It is then I see her. Not Jane this time but someone else, another girl. I happen to glance up and for the briefest of moments I believe I've been flung back to the islands. This girl also skulks along the edge of the corridor, as I have all morning, her black skin a shadow among white faces. She wears no matching sweater-and-skirt set. Her plaid blouse tugs tight across her shoulders, the cuffs too small to be buttoned. But her skin, yes, I feel as if her skin has surely been warmed by tropical suns. Her skin, her beautiful black skin, reminds me of the islands and I smile.

"Hi," I say to her. I introduce myself.

She stops walking. She says nothing, staring at me as if she's not sure I'm in my right senses. I tell her I'm new and ask if she'll eat with me. She shrugs and glances around the corridor as if searching for someone with whom she thinks I would rather eat. But then she looks back, her eyes slightly lowered, suspicious perhaps. "Yeah, I guess," she says, shrugging again, still not smiling. "Those yours?" She nods toward my books and jacket, then asks for my combination: She understands I can't open the locker. She opens it for me, shows me how to do it, and I pile my stuff inside. Then I follow her down the corridor to the cafeteria.

After waiting in the lunch line, not speaking—neither of us can think of anything to say—I follow her to the farthest corner of the cafeteria. I understand she sits here alone every day, and now we will sit here alone together, as if we are shunned. I place my tray across from hers and stare at the frank and beans, at the carton of milk. Still we have trouble speaking. She seems so shy I'm even afraid to ask her name, but finally I do. She tells me, "Betty."

That's all. As if there isn't any reason why I would want to know her last name or anything else about her.

She asks me where I live. I don't want to tell her, am embarrassed to tell her. I know, from driving around Glen Rock, that I live in the newest and most expensive section of town. "Lowell Road," I say softly, hoping the name of the street will mean nothing to her.

But she nods and tells me her mother works as a maid in lots of those pretty houses. She says this almost proudly, as if it's an accomplishment to work in a pretty house, or she is proud of her mother. I am the one embarrassed—not for her, no, but for myself. I think of our wall-to-wall carpeting, the large kitchen with breakfast room, the wood-paneled dining room, the fireplace, the two baths, all our new furniture, new bedspreads, new drapes. I don't want this house, this closet full of new Stateside clothes. I know what we have is too much, even though our possessions never seem to be enough for my parents.

The blonde girl, with a small group of friends, enters the cafeteria. I lean forward in my chair—I must—as if this will allow them to notice me. I want them to see me, walk over to me, select me for a friend. They don't. What can I do? What can I say? Who can I be? I don't know the language, the magic, of these beautiful, well-behaved, well-scrubbed girls who live in New Jersey suburbs. Yes, for years these girls *have* been scrubbed in warm, sudsy New Jersey shower water, while I, in St. Thomas, was cleansed in sun and in the salty sea—which I'd thought was cleansing. Now, looking at these girls, I see I am wrong. For the bright colors of the tropics—all that I know—look garish here in this clean, white cafeteria. If these girls even dare glance my way, their eyes will quickly turn from me as if my body has been bathed forever in the wrong color, in the wrong light.

"That's Jane Johnson," Betty says.

She's followed my gaze and I look back at her, embarrassed. She understands she is not my first choice of lunch partners.

"Who're the others?"

Robin Hays, Ginger Walker, Vicki Sheldon, Elizabeth Parker. Their names are listed, first and last. "They get all the good grades and all the boys like them."

The next morning I don't want to return to school. I sit on my bed clasping my zippered notebook.

"Is Jane Johnson a Jewish name?" I ask my mother when she comes to see if I'm ready. I am looking for a connection.

"No," she says. "Why? What's the matter?"

"I don't look like them, like the others," I say. "That's the matter."

"You look very nice, dear."

I know I don't. Because I don't look Christian—or as if I were raised in New Jersey—I know I could never look nice and that none of these girls will ever like me. "Besides," I say, "I'm too old to wear my hair in a stupid ponytail. I want to cut it off."

My mother sits beside me, but makes no move to touch my hand or comfort me. Her words are measured and definite: "Your hair's fine. You know how your father loves it." She whisks a stray strand from my neck. "Believe me, you're not too old for a ponytail. There's no need to look sophisticated for schoolboys. There's only one thing they want. You stay away from them or you'll get yourself pregnant."

I'd been staring at the blue rug next to the bed. Slowly, I begin to glance up at my mother as if, by seeing her eyes, I'll truly be able to understand what she just said. My gaze rises up to her waist, her shoulder, her chin—but then quickly I glance away, believing it too dangerous for us to look at each other, too dangerous for me to know what she meant.

"Honey, cheer up. You look fine. Soon as everyone gets to know you, they'll like you. Just give it some time," she says.

But there is no time. I want to look Christian now. I want to be a New Jersey girl now. I want to molt my tropical skin to a cool shade of winter. I must. For how can I return to school until I decipher the secret language of New Jersey suburbs, until I learn the magic of ordinary New Jersey towns, houses, streets?

□ □ □

Every morning, on the way to school, my sister and I sit in the back seat of the black Fleetwood Cadillac the bank has bought my father. I am embarrassed by this car, too. Jane's mother brings her to school in a cream-colored station wagon, and I want that car, wish we had a practical cream-colored station wagon, a sturdy family car. Surely if you drive a sturdy family car you will have a practical, sturdy family. And Jane's mother, I also notice, is neatly dressed and energetic. She does not remind me of the mothers in St. Thomas who sleep and drink in the afternoons behind closed hurricane shutters. I believe Jane must have inherited her own neatness and energy from her mother. And perhaps I almost understand a small connection between mothers and daughters, between fathers and daughters. But no—I am not ready to know.

During the drive to school my father tells my sister and me about his work, the success of the bank. Neither she nor I respond, but we know no response is necessary. Simply, he needs to tell us, even though, over the years, he will never notice that my sister and I don't listen. Over the years I will smile to myself when I see my sister drift beyond the reach of his voice. Out of the corner of my eye I watch her now. *Kiki,* I whisper to myself. I want to ask her to walk me to class. I want to ask her to hold my hand and guide me through school. But she ignores me the way she ignores our father. She stares out the window, her eyes safely blank. Her mouth is set. Her schoolbooks are neatly stacked in her lap, her hands tightly clasped on top of them. Her fingernails are clean and manicured. Her legs are crossed, hitching up the hem of her plaid skirt. And her pale kneecap, for just that moment, breaks my heart.

The moment the car stops in front of the school, my sister flings open the door and bolts, barely saying good-bye. I leave more slowly, not wanting to hurt my father's feelings. I lean over the seat to kiss him good-bye on the cheek, like any daughter would do. Now, in the morning, his bay rum aftershave is strong and fresh and the scent makes me dizzy. But never in the morning when I arrive at school do I think about what happens at night. Perhaps he doesn't either, for he lightly pats my shoulder and tells me to have a good day. His words are thin; his glance is absent. He's planning his day at the bank now and doesn't need his daughter.

□ □ □

No, Mother. I will not stay away from boys at school. Almost from the start I notice Christopher and want him for my boyfriend. *But you are wrong, Mother.* Certainly *he* doesn't want *that;* if he wanted that, with me, he could have it. I am the one who wants *that.* He sits next to me in English. In his shyness he barely glances at me when I slide into my seat and mumble, "Hello."

□ □ □

I feel contrary—conflicting desires, odd angles that don't fit. First, I am Dina. Silent Dina, who desires nothing for herself. With lowered eyes she sees no one; with her silent mouth she never speaks. When Sue's father fucks Dina she is ordered never to look at his face. She will be hit if she does. But she doesn't. The moment he touches her—no, even before—her eyes are shut tight. She has no need to see what's done to her body because it's not hers. She is not the one who owns it; he does. Dina has the freedom, the luxury, of no responsibility. He does what's necessary to nourish her body, and she will do anything he wants. He doesn't ask. Nor would she want him to. He orders and demands, and she will acquiesce. Her sole role is to serve him, to fulfill any need or desire he might have.

Celeste, however, is usurping Dina: Celeste, with her blonde hair and garnet lips, with ivory skin she wants to see bruised. She wants sexual marks on her body: teeth marks, fingernail marks, blood-kiss marks, fist marks, slap marks, rope marks, belt marks. She wears all these marks proudly, like tattoos. She will look her rapist right in his eyes and dare him. He will punish her for the bold look and she will crave the pain. It nourishes her body and emboldens her. Celeste wants Dina, passive Dina, weak Dina, stone cold dead.

There is me. Then Dina. Then Celeste. From a distance I observe everything they do. But I am not one thing, one entity, either. I am shy and shamed, as I was on the first day of school. I can also hide the shyness and the shame beneath the exterior of a girl who wants to be popular. A girl who wants to be liked. A girl who will do anything, be anything, in order to be liked, anything to obscure the shame of her body.

So, then, all this is me. And more. I am a palimpsest. Erase Celeste. Erase Dina. Erase me—whom I appear to be—and there is yet another girl, a little girl, someone else, but she is the one person I can't see. This little girl is a faint smudge, as transparent as a shadow, her body hiding inside a flower petal, or her heart hidden deep inside a rock. For this little girl must hide. It is far too dangerous for her to come out. Once I caught a glimpse of her running down the beach as I flew away from the island. That was the only time I saw her; I have not seen her since. So how do I know she's still with me? The knowledge is far from conscious. The fact will remain hidden for years. But sometimes, in a total absence of worldly sound, in a stillness as black as the night sky, I hear the faintest of pulses; no, it's not a sound, but I feel, yes, *feel* the faintest of pulses, beating. And the pulse is not mine.

So who wants Christopher? Celeste wants to corrupt him. She wants to unfurl his shyness from his sleeping body and shock it awake. She would teach him everything Sue's father has taught her. Dina, however, will never understand his shyness. Passively, she needs for him to desire her body, the one thing he's most unable to do. Since this is how she believes she is loved, she will never believe he cares for her, loves her.

I, on the other hand, desire his shyness, that he barely notices my body. I love his scent of white soap, the way he smells when I slide past him to reach my desk. From the corner of my eye, as I try to listen to the teacher, I see his clean fingernails. The palest of hairs on his wrists glisten. I love his small pug nose. And how straight is the part in his clean blonde hair. He looks like no one who could be born into my family.

□ □ □

And now I understand that in order for Christopher to see me *I* must look like no one who could be born into my family. To begin, I chop off my hair. Except I botch it badly, and my angry mother refuses to take me to a beauty parlor to salvage what remains. I steal the allowance my sister saved for a new sweater and march to the salon. I tell the beautician to style my hair in a short flip, and teased. All the way home, walking down Main Street, I smile coolly, like Jane. I admire my reflection in store windows and glance to see if anyone I know is inside. And since the beautician has instructed me to set my hair every night, I stop at the drugstore and with the remaining money buy huge pink plastic rollers and a can of Aqua Net hair spray. Tomorrow I will enter the school lobby for the first time with my new hair. Tomorrow, I firmly believe, my new image will reflect the first glimmers of a New Jersey schoolgirl. I want to sit in a chair all night not to disturb my hair, not to crush this image.

Neither my mother nor my sister recognizes this new image. Only my father is the one to tell me I look pretty, tell me I am a beautiful, *his* beautiful, beautiful girl.

It is then I see the mistake. My error. I go to my room, close the door, and sit before the vanity, staring at myself in the mirror. My hair is rigid and sleek from the spray. Not a strand has blown out of place. I look perfect. I need for my hair to look perfect, but he, *he,* I now realize, will disturb the perfection.

When the doorknob turns I barely raise my gaze. In the mirror I watch the door open and my father appear. Softly—the door doesn't even tap—he closes it behind him. He pushes in the button, locking it. I don't turn around. I say nothing. My eyes are now focused on the mirror, but see nothing. I hear him cross the room. I feel him press against me, where I sit on the stool, the back of my head hard against him. He runs his fingers through my perfect hair, brushes it up from my neck, kisses the back of my neck, whispering how beautiful I am with my new hair style. He reaches over and unbuttons my white lacy blouse. If I look in the mirror I will see his hands on my breasts.

But it is only in the mirror where this happens. It must be, since I feel nothing. But then no longer am I even in front of the mirror. I am inside it, trapped in the mirror, hard as glass, and as cold. I feel nothing. I see nothing. It is not possible for me to look back outside. By the time he turns the stool and unzips his fly, Celeste gazes straight into his unsmiling eyes. And right before Celeste bends close to touch him, she smiles into those eyes—knowing this will enrage him. And it does. She wants to feel the fury of his rage. He pushes his penis into her mouth and keeps it there, hard against her throat. And he doesn't stop, he won't stop—her forehead bangs his belt buckle in a thin, tinny sound—he won't stop until she is weeping in fury.

□ □ □

In the center of night, I turn on my light. I wait for this moment when everyone is sleeping. I must. In the center of night, even in winter, my skin smells of sweat, the sheets smell of sweat and of . . . but I can fix this. Yes, I must. Tired, groggy, I stumble to the vanity and sit on the stool, staring dumbly for a moment until I am fully awake. My hair is a mess. Yes, this hair style is a mistake. The ponytail was easier—just yank back the tangles and wind a rubber band around it. No need even to unravel the snarls. But I don't, won't, surrender. I will not let my hair grow long again. The flip stays. Slowly, I urge the comb through my hair—no, the brush first—untangle the big snarls first, then the smaller ones, with the tortoiseshell comb. I curl my hair clump by clump, layer by layer, fastening the rollers with silver clips. I tie a pink net over the rollers and spray it with Aqua Net. I learn to crave the scent of Aqua Net. I spray more than is necessary and will spray even more on my hair in the morning, this Aqua Net, covering all other smells on my body. Then I dress for school. Slip. Skirt. Bra. Blouse. Socks. I put a gold circle pin on my collar. Carefully I lie back in bed, pull up the covers, sleep a few more hours, ready for school in the morning.

□ □ □

In the eighth grade I buy a big box of Christmas cards and send a card to every girl I want for my friend, as well as a few boys, including Christopher. I do this in secret since my mother would be outraged by this overt display of Christianity. I mail the cards early to ensure there will be time for everyone to mail me a card back. I receive lots back and display them like trophies: on the bookcase, on the dresser, on my desk, on the vanity. Over and over I read the printed Hallmark messages, as if the messages were written just for me.

As the days near Christmas, I still have not received a card from Jane or from Christopher. I meet the mailman at the front door. From sitting next to Christopher in English class, I know his handwriting, and I quickly flip through the mail. Finally, on December 24, I receive a card from him. It is from a large boxed set of cards such as mine. There is no special note below his signature. It is signed simply "Christopher." I rush to my room, close the door, and rub my finger over and over his blue-inked name. No card arrives from Jane, but I will try again next year.

□ □ □

I sit before my gym locker slowly tying my sneakers. I untie the laces, then tie them again. I delay undressing, hoping most of the girls will change quickly and go out to the gym. I pull off my sweater and unbutton my blouse, trying to hide behind the small locker door. As usual my green gym suit is dirty and wrinkled. It's supposed to be starched and ironed, but I never remember to bring it home to wash it. I have trouble with showers and clean clothes, overwhelmed by the enormity, the impossible job, of keeping myself clean, feeling defeated before I even begin. As a child in Washington I felt comforted by folding my handkerchiefs and arranging my Monday, Tuesday, Wednesday underwear in bureau drawers. Now, my bureau is in disarray. My clothes are in disarray. I am in disarray. There doesn't seem to be time to keep gym suits clean or clothes ironed. Quickly I slip into my suit and snap the buttons.

In the gym I lie on the mat with the other girls warming up, stretching, doing sit-ups, push-ups. My body performs the exercises smoothly. This is important. I must be good in gym. My body doesn't want to be singled out for inadequacy. My body must perform perfectly—and besides, Robin, Jane's friend, is in my gym class, so I must be noticed and admired.

Four ropes hang across the width of the gym. I have never climbed ropes before, so I wait at the end of the line, watching the other girls, studying their movements. When it is my turn I grip the rope in my hands, wind it between my legs, clamp it between my feet, and pull. A heavy girl beside me struggles, but I don't feel sorry for her—I can't. I can't afford to feel sorry. I must be the best in my group, or at least as good as the best. Another girl moves faster than I toward the top, but this isn't so much a race as it is endurance: just make it to the top and down again, gracefully. I must. I maintain my form, the way our gym teacher taught us, inching upward. I glance toward the ceiling. I'm halfway there. I must touch that spot of white paint, leave a mark, before I can come back down. Only a handful of girls who preceded me reached the top—Robin, of course, was one. When she'd finished I'd warmly congratulated her, admired her form, ingratiating myself—as I must. She must like me. When I glance down I see her watching me.

The heavy girl droops to the bottom. She sits on the mat rubbing her hands, staring at them, embarrassed. Even though my palms burn, I continue. I will make it to the top even if all the skin on my palms blisters. I clamp the rope between my feet and push, my arms pull, I take a deep breath. The other girl has reached the top and is now sliding down, the rope a bit loose between her legs, using her arms more than her legs, but she'll be all right. The fourth girl struggles below me; I don't think she'll make it.

With a surge, my fingertips sweep the ceiling. Below, there is a smattering of applause and my heart races. I know I'm grinning, can't stop grinning, and I even linger at the top, plant my palm flat to the ceiling, push against it, swaying in the slow motion of the rope.

With perfect form I lower myself, my arms and legs steady, still in control. When my sneakers hit the mat, a few girls congratulate me, including Robin, with her shiny hair, sparkling brown eyes, dazzling smile. I am thrilled—and still grinning. As we move to the pommel horse, *I* go first now, the first girl in line, not needing to wait to watch others. I run, run down the floor toward the springboard, my eyes focused, my sneakers pounding up the short ramp. A big bounce on the board and I'm sailing, till my hands grip the handles, my legs spread in perfect form, yes, I can feel the parts of my body perfectly placed and balanced, and I'm flying again, now over the horse, free of the horse toward the mat, my eyes open wide—and alive.

Back in the locker room I laugh and joke with the girls. *The shower will be all right. I will be all right.* We kick off our sneakers and gossip about boys, gossip about teachers. Complain about homework. I agree with everything anyone says. As we move to the showers I hold my small white towel loosely in front of my body like everyone else. We are all the same. We hang our towels on hooks and enter. I must enter. The shower is a small tiled room, sprays attached to the walls and to a pole in the center. I must act as if I'm all right. I am here/not here. I don't feel the spray but I see it, see beads of water on my skin, hear nothing, do not hear girls' voices, only a throb. I must circle the room completely before exiting by the same door. I do this, although I don't pause before a spray to soap myself as I'm supposed to. I hurry out and grab my towel, quickly dressing. But no one has said anything about my body. I'm okay. I wasn't noticed.

Then it's the most natural thing—a group of girls heads toward the cafeteria. I am with them, along with Robin, swept along on giggles and surefooted movements on these once-tricky, mazy corridors. I expect to find myself alone when we reach the cafeteria, but still I am awash in their flow of words. And there I am at the same table as Jane. Not next to her, but at the fringes, and she has smiled at me—*smiled*—and I bask in the warm stream of girl-words.

But there is Betty, alone in her corner—what had been *our* corner—huddled over her food. We do not have the same classes, and I had forgotten to meet her by the bulletin board in the lobby. She does not glance at me, not once, but I am certain she saw me rushing through the lobby. I know she saw me or else she would have waited. I also know I can't invite her over to join me. My own status at this table is too shaky.

I put down the fork. I am no longer hungry. I no longer hear the girls' chatter. As much as I know I can't invite Betty here, I also know I can't afford to leave here and join her, though she would never have joined the girls at this table without me. She would never have abandoned me alone to the corner.

The next morning while sitting before the mirror I notice, for the first time, that my island tan has faded. My skin is almost as pale as Jane's and Robin's. No longer do I dream of crimson sunsets. My saddle-shoed feet are beginning to understand the rigidly blocked sidewalks of suburban New Jersey streets.

□ □ □

I learn Christopher's schedule. Between classes I place myself where we will either have to pass each other in the hall or walk in the same direction. Always, I smile. It is always returned. I've learned he does not have a girlfriend. This endless preoccupation enables me to forget, forget, forget . . .

The eighth-grade class has a Spring Fling. Pink rollers have been in my hair since morning, and at 6:30 I unwind them, comb my hair, tease the bangs into place. I spray Aqua Net and study my face in the mirror. I rearrange a strand or two and drink a bottle of 7-Up—dinner—a 7-Up is enough for dinner. I slip into my white dress with small pink flowers and apply pink lipstick. I dab White Rose Petroleum Jelly on my eyebrows and lashes. I want to wear eye makeup, and decide to buy some with my next allowance. I study my reflection, try different expressions. Friendly. Sultry. Indifferent. Bored. When I part my lips and lean close to the mirror, I see a flicker of an expression I don't recognize. I touch the mirror as if to stop—hold—the look—*Who are you?* But she is gone.

In the living room my father reads the *New York Times*. I pause before him waiting for a compliment, wanting him to tell me I look pretty for my first school dance. He does not look up from the newspaper. He does not say good-bye.

In the car, my mother and I are silent. I sit in the back seat watching the town out the window as lights in all the houses are switched on. I wonder what it would be like if I wandered inside a stranger's house. I wonder what *I* would be like if I lived in one of these other houses, had another home, a different name, different parents. I imagine sitting down to dinner with a different family, and the father would talk to me about . . . but I can't think of what. What do fathers say to daughters? What? Tell me, tell me, tell me: *Daddy, tell me something.* I'm scared there is nothing to say.

I meet my girlfriends in the lobby. Walking down the hall to the cafeteria we chatter, pretending we are just going for lunch. But surely we all look pretty, in our better-than-school-dress dresses, with our pink fingernail polish, with our scents of floral perfumes, all different, like a bouquet. We duck into the girls' room and line up before the mirror. We help to groom each other, not *for* each other, but for the boys, checking for stray hairs or smudged lipstick. I pray I will not be the only girl not asked to dance, pray Christopher will ask me to dance. I wonder what I must do to ensure this happens.

As a disc jockey spins records, girls with the softest of cheeks and lotioned hands, boys with the frailest of down on their cheeks and sports-roughened hands test the music, the romance. The girls seem assured, seem to understand the movements of the dance, and I worry I lack their confidence and grace, that I will not be the girl Christopher searches for. I remember the dance in St. Thomas, the dance with the sailors on the *Danmark*. If Christopher notices Dina . . . if—but no, Celeste would never come to this dance.

When I see Christopher at the refreshment table, I wander over and pick up a cup of red punch. I smile, he smiles, and now I believe I'll be okay, that I can be the girl, any girl Christopher would like for me to be, yes, I will be her as soon as I understand whom he wants to see when he looks at me. We talk about classes, the wrestling season just ended, the baseball season beginning. He's on the team, he tells me, and I say I'll watch him play, pretending to love baseball, although I've never seen a game. He says that's great, that he has four younger sisters who hate it, and thought all girls hated sports.

"That's a lot of sisters," I say.

He nods. "They're great, but they can be a real handful."

"Like how?" I say.

"You name it. There's always a lot of faces to wash and a lot of teeth to brush." He smiles. "I single-handedly taught all four to tie their shoelaces."

"Gosh," I say. "You must be a cool older brother."

Finally he invites me to dance. He's only a few inches taller than I, so I can clearly see his round green eyes, their soft expression, as if he doesn't have any secrets. From the way this shy young boy holds my hand and carefully touches my back, I think of the way these hands must gently wash his sisters' faces, tie their laces. I wonder what it must be like to be one of his sisters, a little girl with freshly scrubbed cheeks and sparkling teeth, eyes like her brother. I try to imagine, imagine her . . . until I begin to feel I might almost *be* her, begin to feel that I am pitching backward to a time . . . falling backward to a place I can only think of as "before." And I would not have been able to say *before what*, exactly. Just before. All I know is that, with Christopher, my body feels shy in his shy arms, my hand feels shy in the foreignness of *his* kind of boy-man hands. Except as the record ends and he quickly releases my hand, I begin to worry I could never be one of his sisters—or *like* his sisters. So surely the shyness must be Christopher's; it must be his sisters'. It isn't mine. And I know the longer we stand beside each other, the more I feel I should warn him. *Stay away, Christopher. I can destroy you.* I know what Celeste can do. But he doesn't hear the warning.

Shortly before ten I go outside to wait for my mother. A spring drizzle dampens the air, and I stand beneath the overhang watching headlights. Behind one of the pillars I notice a movement, a boy kissing a girl. I can barely see them, but still I imagine her back pressed against the pillar, his body pressed against hers. I almost take a step toward them, wanting . . . What? No, it isn't me who wants. It's *her.* Celeste. The other "me." She senses—how can she not?—senses the pressure of his lips. She knows this pressure, understands it far better than I understand Christopher. Perhaps they hear me—I don't know—but the girl pushes the boy away. He struggles with her, not wanting to let go, but she pushes again and he releases her.

Ryan. He's in my class, but I don't know the girl. Her smudged mouth looks scared. Her eyes are lowered as she rushes past me. I stare straight at Ryan, except the gaze doesn't seem to be mine—that expression I'd glimpsed in the mirror earlier—it's too direct for an eighth grader. And I smile at him with a mouth that is far from scared, with a mouth that says: I am not the kind of girl who would push you away. He seems startled, pauses for a moment, uncertain what is meant, perhaps. As he passes he brushes the edge of my dress.

In my bedroom I turn off the lights and open the window to the spring rain. The lilacs just below my window smell like wet, dusky shadows. These lilacs. The scent stays with me every day, even in winter. The pale lavender color twines with the heavy, dripping scent. In these lilacs I feel the gentleness of nature as well as its danger. I understand that Christopher's innocence is fear—but that Ryan's danger is also fear, and that by being opposites they are really opposite sides of the same scared boy. And that I, I am the one who will always scare them.

□ □ □

I lie in bed. Sprinklers cool green summer lawns up and down Lowell Road. Every Saturday morning mowers whir the silence of neatly trimmed houses and flower beds. My father spends hours killing crabgrass and weeds. Our yard must look as perfect as other yards; our house will look as perfect as other houses. *We* will look perfect—as perfect as my beautiful baby-blue bedroom with matching curtains and ruffled bedspread. Behind the lids of my eyes I sense sunlight rimming the curtains. I don't want to open them yet: my eyes or the curtains. Inside, the house is quiet. Our grandmother has moved to a nursing home about an hour away, and my mother visits her Saturdays. Surely my sister, an early riser, has disappeared for the day.

I've done little this summer except read. The kids from school don't call, and I am too shy to call them, afraid they won't remember me or won't want to hear from me. I've bought a new swimsuit, but have not gone to the public pool where most of the kids will be. Really, I'd rather read.

So once a week, when I receive my allowance, I take the bus from Glen Rock to the bookstore in Ridgewood. There, I spend hours browsing. I am nearly breathless as my hand opens the door, breathless for that first moment when my feet touch the uneven, old wood floor. It is scuffed from shoes, scarred from the passage of the ladder needed to reach books up near the ceiling. It's as if the shoes and the ladder have worn away layers of wood down to its essence, an essence that smells warm, smooth, safe. I am full of the scent of inked paper on the rows and rows of books, full of the feel of the thin layer of dust on the books on the upper shelves. I rub the dust between thumb and forefinger. The books are arranged neatly, their spines straight and identified by title and author. Surely my hand nearly trembles as I reach for a certain book. And when I see beautiful covers, pictures of oceans and fields, cities of today or cities of faraway times and places—in red, yellow, green ink—I must sit on a carton of unpacked books or on the bottom rung of the ladder to study them. All these books remind me of my Uncle Esey's study. I miss my Uncle Esey. My mother and her sister had a fight, and we never see my aunt and uncle anymore, but I feel closer to him here, surrounded by shelves of books.

I read *Anna Karenina, Lord Jim, The Sound and the Fury, Crime and Punishment, The Idiot, The Brothers Karamazov, Grapes of Wrath, How Green Was My Valley, The Once and Future King, The Scarlet Letter, Heart of Darkness, Jane Eyre, Wuthering Heights, To Kill a Mockingbird, The Member of the Wedding, Huckleberry Finn, The Ballad of the Sad Café*. Some novels I understand better than others, but that hardly matters. To be reading words, to be seeing images, to be characters in novels, to be in their houses and towns and cities, to be in their lives, to *be* their lives, is what matters. It is the books themselves that matter: to be able to hold these worlds, these words, these characters, in the palms of my hands. To lie on my bed and, when I finish a novel, to be able to press the open pages of the novel against my face and smell the words, the lives, the cities, the towns, the characters, their wishes and desires, matter. I am not only characters, places, themes, I am the words themselves. These words keep me safe. They are definite, concrete, lasting. No one can take them from me. Rather, *I* am the one who takes, stealing words from these novels like a thief. I hoard words. I collect them. I stuff myself full of them. Not words that bring me closer to reality; rather, words that carry me farther away. I never read books that tell me about my self. Instead, words give me the power to create a person who might be another self, as well as the power to create magical images, a destination, a habitat, where this other self can live.

When I get home from the bookstore I hurry to my bedroom and close the door. I want to lock it—I'm not allowed to—but I treat these books as if they're secrets. I want no one to see them; I want no one to know what I'm reading. I want these books, these characters, these words, to belong to me only, as if no one else in the world has ever read them. I ease the books from the sack and line them on my bed, staring at the covers for hours, before I can possibly decide which one I will choose first to read.

So I lie in bed on a Saturday morning. Early summer heat drifts through raised windows. Without opening my eyes I reach for the book I have placed under the bed. Maybe I will stay in bed all day, reading. I will not leave my room, not even turn on the light, able, even in this gray light, to see the words clearly. But first, under the sheet I hug the book to me, feeling the wedge of pages in my fingers. My fingers search for the dog-ear to determine the distance left before the novel is finished, not wanting any novel ever to be finished. But quickly I'll begin another, as if the first page of *Huckleberry Finn* is the last page of *Anna Karenina*. Perhaps in Huck Finn's adventures he'll discover Anna beneath the train in Russia; perhaps he can even save her. Perhaps it's possible to rearrange worlds and words until things work out better.

The lawnmower stops outside my bedroom window. The sound feels truncated, its cessation louder than the sound itself. I think I feel the air inside the house rush out, think I hear my father breathing outside my bedroom window. I feel the petals of fading lilacs shiver, even think I feel him snap off a cluster—but maybe I only remember he enters my bedroom with a spray of them in a crystal vase which he sets on the headboard as a present.

He smells of mowed grass and sweat. Then a glimpsed memory, a memory of scent—in Washington—his smell of sawdust and raw wood. I try to feel *years,* a connection between years. Who was I then? Who am I now? How does this connect me to back then? My thoughts scatter. He takes the book from my grasp and discards it on my desk, wanting to let me know it's unimportant. He pulls my nightgown over my head, then watches me while he undresses. For *this* is what's important. He is quiet this morning, this early Saturday, as he curls beside me in bed, holding me to his chest, my back against his chest, his lips against my spine where I feel him breathing. He whispers he loves me. I nod, yes, I know that you do, Father, you do. If I can hold this. If we don't move. If we can lie here like this, then I can almost pretend this is love. For years I will try to pretend this, even though he will move. Even though he will, in just a moment, pull my body around, urging me even closer, while we both smell the hot scent of wilting lilac.

This is the connection, what connects me to the years.

□ □ □

Summer nights Jewish kids from Glen Rock, Fair Lawn, and Ridgewood gather at the Jewish Community Center. My mother drives me over, forcing me to go. She tells me I'll have a good time—"You'll see"—and tells me my father will pick me up promptly at 10:30. I don't want to go. I don't want to be with Jewish kids, especially not now while I'm practicing to be Christian. Angry at my mother, I slam the car door, already planning to break all the rules.

I have dressed to break all the rules. I knew the recreation room would be too bright, while the kids, the Cokes, the cookies, would be too boring. So in order to save the evening I've worn red-red shorts, a tight red and white shirt, an apple necklace, and red lipstick. It is the red, of course, that counts. I count on the red to ensure the evening will not be what my mother wants for me. I count on the red to ensure I'll dance with someone, or do something, that isn't boring.

I put a fist on my hip, bend a knee, tilt my head—my interpretation of sophistication—as I watch boys, strangers from other communities. No, I watch one boy, one stranger from another community. He seems older. His sweaty face is unshaven. He's untucked and unironed, his brown, wrinkled shirt hanging carelessly over khaki shorts. He is smoking. Never have I seen a teenager smoke before. So, with him, it is the cigarette that counts. Not just that he's smoking, but that it hangs slack from his mouth. Even if he weren't smoking, I would be able to imagine the cigarette there, as if his full, damp lips would always hold it.

I will him to notice me in the same way I'd willed Ryan to pause that night outside the school dance. He *will* notice me. Steve, this is his name, *will* ask me to dance. And he does—as I knew he would. From the way his hands touch me while we dance, I know they are not like Christopher's. Steve's nails are bitten. The fingertips are raw, needing to be healed, but dangerous with this need, needing a girl to heal them, but not with her small teenage innocent words, innocent glances. His fingers, as we dance, press me hard, as if even now, even here, trying to touch bare skin: hard. I know. He knows me, too, knows I am the only one here who can heal those fingertips, and they desperately need healing.

He teases me about the apple necklace, asks why it's whole, why no one has yet taken a bite. I giggle. Mock shy. My eyes lower, but it is Celeste with the garnet red lips, and, I now realize, Celeste who bought the apple necklace. I believe we both seduce him—how can he stand a chance?: my innocence (he will want to corrupt me); her danger (he will know her boundaries are endless). He tells me he's a senior in high school at Fair Lawn. I tell him I'm almost in ninth grade. He asks if I'm allowed to date older guys. I can't speak. I can't answer him. For a moment I giggle so hard I don't think I can stop.

He whispers that he and his friend have a car. Do I want to go for a ride? Yes. I expect the three of us will sit in the front, but Steve pushes me into the rear. This is all arranged smoothly. I don't see: *They* have arranged this beforehand, *they* have done this before and know the plan.

The windows are open and a thick summer breeze fills the car, this and cigarette smoke. My hair whips my cheeks. I try to straighten it. He says: What does it matter? And, of course, it doesn't. For even as he says this, he's pulling me onto his lap. He starts slow, nuzzling my face with his mouth before kissing me, the first man who's kissed me besides my father. At first I'm exhilarated, free with the movement of the car, the first time I'm alone in a car with a boy, free, as if I'm floating far beyond the walls of my house, where no one in my family can touch me, where no one can bring me back. I feel as if this is a rescue, and I am giddy with flight.

His hand is beneath my shorts, those raw fingertips seeking comfort. I look up and see his friend glance at us in the rearview mirror. His glass-cold gaze knows the truth and quickly I close my eyes, not wanting to see it. Steve edges me down on the seat to unzip my shorts. I do not think to struggle. His fingers need me too bad—I know this—as much as I know I will be able to heal them, just as I heal my father.

His friend parks the car. Through the window I hear the friction of a thousand night insects rubbing their legs, filling a field with sound. Yet I can't smell the field, instead smell the plastic seat of the car. Steve's sweat. Cigarette smoke. His need. The car gently rocks as his friend leaves it. And Steve is whispering, whispering how good it feels, how much he loves this, how much he needs *this*. Yes, of course, I have always known this, long before I knew him. He does not use the pronoun "you." He doesn't need me. It is *this, this, this* that pushes my thighs to the seat. He needs this. I whisper that I love him. I have been trained to say this. But I believe I mean it, even though I don't know his last name.

I don't need to know his last name. I know him anyway. Driving here I'd felt as if I were finally free, far away from home. Now I understand I've gone nowhere. So, yes, without knowing Steve's last name, I know him. Sweat from his face drips on mine; it is this I know. He pulls himself out and ejaculates onto my stomach; it is this I also know. I know him well enough to understand that when he is finished, when his need is finished, he will be gone. They all will be gone. I will never see him again. Even my father is gone when he finishes, only returning when he needs me.

It is way past 10:30 when they drive me back to the center. My father is not in front. He has not waited. Walking home, I pretend I could be any girl. I *am* any New Jersey girl walking home from a date, any New Jersey girl whose parents will be angry she will be home late, angry she has broken the rules. My father, who is always watching out for me, always watching me, will know what I did tonight and with whom I did it. Since he already knows, since he already knows why he should be angry, I walk slowly through dark neighborhoods under drooping limbs of maples. There is no reason to hurry. It will happen whether I am home now or hours later. Where Steve ejaculated, my shirt sticks to my stomach, and I know I should clean myself before reaching home. But there is no place to stop on these streets. Besides, I know I wouldn't stop. I know what must happen when I reach home. And I know I deserve it.

But I am not the one who deserves it. *She* is the one who deserves it. So I am not any girl, after all. Nor am I just one girl. How lucky, I am several. For the molecules of our several bodies, the molecules of our skin, are imbricated like scales connecting us together. And so I must remember only one of these girls just committed a sin against her father. Just one girl broke the rules and will be punished. Not the others.

Our porch light is on, the only light on the street. The neighbors are asleep, yet as I climb to the top of the stoop and pause in the light, I feel as if they all watch me. And I want them to, *yes, you, I want you to see my shame.* As my mother sees my shame. She yanks me inside and slaps me across the face. I am slapped on my head, breasts, arms, stomach, neck. I am a slut. A whore. No man will marry me. I will get pregnant and disgrace her, disgrace our family. *Yes, Mother, you are right,* I think. All this will happen. I notice she had been sleeping in the living room, on the couch, while she waited. And I realize he is alone at the back of the house in his bedroom. Or mine. It is my sister who was awarded the master bedroom, the only room upstairs. She sleeps alone, separate from the rest of us. My mother—my mother tells me I won't be allowed outside for the rest of the summer. I am grateful. For how wrong I was to betray my father, and I must be kept safe from all danger outside this house. My mother turns from me. Perhaps tonight she will continue to sleep here on the couch. Yes. She will allow my father and me the privacy of the back bedroom.

This is where he has come to wait. We are alone in my bedroom, the door locked. He takes off my clothes and sees, or touches, Steve's dried semen on my stomach. Or perhaps he smells it even before I reach the bedroom. I believe he smelled me as I still walked home down the street. Surely the smell of Steve is all over me: his semen, his cigarette smoke, his sweat, his touch. His fingerprints tattoo my body. Enraged, my father pushes me down on the bed. He screams at me, yet I don't hear words, only sounds. He grips the chain of my necklace and holds it tight against my neck. He seems confused. He doesn't know what to do with me. He begins to fuck me, stops. He's too angry. No, he won't touch me there, not until it's been punished. He will punish it until it is his again. He yanks open my bureau drawers until he finds nylon stockings. He ties down my arms and legs, restraining me. *But don't you know, Father, you don't have to do this? I won't resist. I won't refuse. I refuse you nothing, Father.*

On my desk is an empty 7-Up bottle and he jams the cool impersonal glass into me. His rage wants to jam it up, up into my stomach, and when he can't he heaves the bottle against the wall with such force it shatters. With a piece of glass he starts to cut me, down there. It etches my skin almost neatly, razor thin, precise, and so, so cool against my blood that I shiver. I feel it perfectly. *Yes, cut me, Father. I want to bleed. Let us bleed together, bleed this everlasting evil from our bodies.* I believe I relish the scent of blood, the warmth of it dripping between my thighs. He punctures my nipples with his fingernails, until they bleed, too, and I welcome this, all of this. This ritual to cleanse my body will make me his again. I want to be his. *Yours, Father. I will always belong to you, Father. Forgive me.*

There is only one way he can forgive me. He smears White Rose Petroleum Jelly on himself and rapes my bottom. I watch blood drip on the already bloody sheet, and I welcome this, all of this. There is something wrong with me, he says, I am a nymphomaniac, and although I don't know what the word means, I nod my head, agreeing. He says I need help, I need more, I need it so badly, and he, *he,* is the only one who can help me. He goes to the kitchen and returns with another bottle, an empty. This, I know he believes, will console me. If only he could keep it inside me forever, not just this one long night. But now, yes, I am his again. And I know and I know I am forgiven.

I think it is morning. I measure time by his rage, which explodes and subsides, explodes and subsides. I can no longer tell whether I'm tied, but it doesn't matter. For this is where I belong. I know it. Outside the window the girl who lives next door plays, but surely I pity her and don't want to join her. Over and over, Donna's tricycle clacks up and down her drive just outside my bedroom window, until the sound rattles my skull—while inside my bedroom my father fucks me—until there is no longer a me. For it's not true that a body is needed, like a jar, to contain everything inside it. There is a stain on the sheet that is an essence of me, but there is no tangible me. And if there were a me who could go outside . . . if there were a me who could watch Donna ride her tricycle . . . But I can't go outside. I wouldn't go outside even if my father released me. And we both know he can't.

□ □ □

It is September. It is the first day of school, my last year of junior high. I wear a freshly pressed white Oxford shirt with a button-down collar. I wear an autumn-colored vest with matching skirt. Such lovely new clothes my mother bought me, such a pretty outfit. My face and body are scrubbed, my hair shampooed, worn in a ponytail again after growing long over the summer. Now I am numb again, like that other first day: from the voices of students, from the clang of lockers, from the smell of chalk dust. I move slowly. As I shuffle along the corridor, I believe I'm just learning to walk. Someone says, "Hi." I smile, about to speak, but no sound comes from my mouth. For a moment I think I am drowning.

□ □ □

For months I drag my body to school and home, school and home. No longer does it seem to carry me. I think I sit with JaneRobin-VickieElizabeth at lunch, but I don't remember. And no longer does it matter. In the halls I pass Christopher and we smile, but he seems to have drifted away. Nights and mornings are cool with frost, and it seems to speckle my skin's surface. I long for winter. I long for rock-solid ground upon which to walk. I long for trees encased in sheaths of ice, for the frigid, deadening air of winter. During class I look outside—not that I long to be there, on the other side of the window. Truly, it doesn't matter where I am. Here. There. I have forgotten how to listen. I want to listen to the teacher, but I can't. My ears are already stuffed full of sound and can hold no more. My mouth is packed full and can hold few words. I am too tired to speak, and sometimes I'm not sure if I'm awake or sleeping. I've almost stopped eating, but the thinner I get, the heavier I feel, until I think I'm dragging dense weight.

A thin autumn sun seeps through the windows of our house. Outside, my father rakes leaves. Sometimes my sister and I help. Other times I sit in the window watching him. Up and down the street, men rake leaves into neat piles, men in plaid flannel shirts and brown corduroy slacks. Next door, Donna will rush at a pile of leaves and jump in it, shouting, her blonde hair streaming past her shoulders. I think I used to do this when we lived in Washington and Maryland. Smoke from chimneys curls into a slow gray sky. The air smells of red smoldering leaves.

In the kitchen my mother bakes a chicken for supper. We will sit around the kitchen table, our family. My father talks about work. His three girls listen. Or pretend to listen. Or perhaps not even pretend. No, I will at least pretend, but it won't matter because he doesn't notice the difference. My elbows rest on the table as I cut my chicken into tiny pieces. It is dry and hard. I think about trying to get enough of it into my mouth. My mother's gaze slides from plate to plate, noticing the intake, whether my father, sister, and I are eating. Whether we eat enough. She wants to fill us with food. Food is all she can give us, her only offering of what she wants to be love. She wants us to eat until we feel stuffed. *Mother, don't you understand? I am already stuffed.* And yet, there will never be enough to truly fill me, fill any of us.

After dinner I lie on my bed. No longer do I sit at my desk to study. No longer do I truly study. Sometimes I stare at my history book for hours—same page, same paragraph, same sentence—until it loops senselessly around my brain without comprehension. I switch on my transistor radio and listen to rock 'n' roll. Even with music, I barely comprehend the lyrics. I want to sit at my desk and study like my sister. I want the energy of my sister, but just watching her makes me tired. I don't know what this noise is in my brain. I try to stop my brain long enough to see it. I try to focus on one clear thought. I can't. Inside my skull there is static and I am without means to silence it. It keeps me awake at night and restless during the day. And yet I know—don't I know?—that if it did stop long enough I wouldn't want to know, I wouldn't want to see what's inside my head. I wouldn't be able to stand it.

My father comes in my room and shuts the door. It is too early, I think. Usually he doesn't come here until everyone is sleeping.

He snuggles beside me and takes the book from my hands. This is fine. I'd never be able to read it. He switches off the radio. This is fine, too, for even if I don't understand the lyrics, I know all the songs are sad. He pulls me to him, tonight smelling of autumn, not bay rum aftershave. Tonight not smelling of the tropics. But what is he doing, who is he, in these new scents he's wearing? He strokes my hair, my shoulders, my face, places he usually forgets to touch. My mother walks down the hall toward the bedrooms, but neither of us stiffens or flinches. She goes into her own bedroom and shuts the door. In a moment she will switch on the radio next to her bed and leave it playing while she waits for the news. My father turns me around till I face him. Quickly I close my eyes, for we never, never see each other. If I open my eyes while he's fucking me, I watch him never once watching my face. He stares down the length of my body to see what he does to it, for he is entranced by what he does. Now, I feel his eyes on my face and I don't know why he has to stare at me now as he strokes my cheeks and the sides of my neck. "I love you so much, my most precious angel," he whispers. His touch is gentle. Loving. Caring. But my face burns in his gaze.

Stop it, Father, I think.

More than anything I want him to stop. *Don't stroke my face, don't whisper that you love me unless you are fucking me.* For I feel as if I'm about to weaken in some unredeemable way. I want to scream to him to stop. To fuck me instead. Hurt me. Surely that is safer than this.

And then I feel it, for the first time, the fist in my throat loosening. I try to swallow it back down but the force is enormous, the force of a fist pushing a foreign moisture, wet and salty, up the stem of my throat till it's about to drip from my eyes. My body is about to convulse. My teeth chatter. I try to clamp them to stop the tears—for they will kill me. Still I feel him stare—and gently, gently, he's stroking my cheeks like a father, stroking the tears away, comforting me, until I feel as if my entire body might be warm, comfortable, vulnerable, and I want to once again feel the safety, the rigidity, of that ice-cold fist—but he is warming me, the skin on his hands healing who I am, and who I *really* am is rising, rising and I must, must, must will her back down. It is not safe for her here. The girl. The girl on the beach, the girl I saw as the plane flew from the island over the Caribbean, the girl I *had* to leave behind. *It is not safe for you here. I'm not ready. Go back. He doesn't mean this,* I warn her. *I must swallow you and you must hide beneath the deepest shadow cast by my heart.* The tears, I fear, will wash her from my eyes. She will be unable to hide and he will gently singe the skin off her body with the rubbing of his hands. Her hair will ignite in the friction of his stroking fingers. But the tears are coming. I beg him: *Stop.* I think I'm screaming. *Father, please, Daddy, just fuck me.* I open my eyes and he smiles.

□ □ □

Once, years later, I see Steve again. I am home from college during Christmas break, shopping at Bambergers in Paramas Mall. There he is, behind the counter, selling men's cologne. At first I simply stare at him, pleased I'm wearing my Boston University sweatshirt, for I'm sure he'd have thought I wouldn't make it to college. While I need no men's cologne—and had just been passing through the department—I approach the counter and ask for a bottle of English Leather. Other than that, we do not speak. I don't know if he recognizes me, but I think not. There is no flicker of recognition in his eyes. When he hands me the change, I see the wounded stubs of his fingers. He has found no one or nothing to permanently heal them. When I get home I feel sad. I don't know what I would have done if he'd asked me to go with him in his car again. I don't know. I open the bottle of English Leather and dab some on my wrists. Every day I do this until the bottle is empty.

□ □ □

In ninth-grade history class I'm asked what I think about the Boston Tea Party. Everyone is asked. Mr. Hall goes around the room asking our opinions. I slump low in my chair. My heart is racing. *Please, please don't ask me.* I never raise my hand in class and I never speak voluntarily. He calls on me. I have the book open to the section and I begin to quote from it. Gently, he tells me to close it, that he knows what the book says; he wants to know what *I* say. What do I think? I think nothing. I don't know what I think. I tell him this, surprised by my boldness. I have no opinion, I say. Who would want to know what *I* think of the Boston Tea Party? He says *he* wants to know what I think. I'm confused. I shake my head, uncertain. He is not trying to shame me. His voice is gentle. I don't want to disappoint him, but I have nothing to say, am too scared to speak, or even to think. What is the Boston Tea Party? I never knew I was allowed to have opinions; no one had ever taught me to think. Almost, almost, something else nudges the rim of my mind . . . *what do I think?* I look up at Mr. Hall, at his brown eyes waiting for me, not trying to rush me. What do I think? Could I tell him? I have never spoken to this man, never been alone with him, never even thought about him, not once, ever. Why do I think there is something more urgent than the Boston Tea Party that I must tell him? "Mr. Hall . . . " My voice is a whisper. He leans toward me, listening. I grip the edge of my desk. But I can't think.

I don't know how to listen to my mind. It is hopeless. There is no word to explain what has just nudged my mind.

□ □ □

Robin's Christmas party, which Christopher attends with me, smells of pine and cinnamon candles. An orange-blue fire in the fireplace warms the living room. On the mantel is a crèche. Carefully, I touch the miniature lambs, touch baby Jesus's head. I stand before the Christmas tree enchanted by red, green, white, gold lights, bubbles of light, reflecting on metallic balls and shivering strands of tinsel. Balls depict scenes of red sleighs filled with people in white furry clothes and scenes of reindeer and Santa Claus. On top, a feathery angel, attached to a star, almost touches the ceiling. Beneath the tree are presents wrapped with bows and Christmas paper.

I believe, more than anything, this is what our family needs: a decorated pine tree placed before the window in our living room. If we had one, how would it be possible to rage at each other? The thin glass ornaments would shatter; no one would want to shatter them. We would have to walk on tiptoe, so the tinsel wouldn't slide from the boughs. If we had a crèche on our mantel, we would have to be careful not to wake the sleeping Jesus.

But we will have no tree or crèche. Nor will we celebrate Chanuka. We have no Menorah or candles. Our family is without ceremony or myth to connect us to a life larger than our own existence. We are without comfort or means to ease the journey, deepen it past the parameters of our house. My sister and I will receive gifts, yes, but they will be given without significance or meaning. They will be worth only the price paid. I want to live in this house with Robin.

Christopher and I dance. All the couples dance, as the bubbles of light on the tree warm us. I inhale the scent of his wool sweater, unused to boys who smell of winter. As each record ends he releases my hand, but we stand together, waiting for the next record. Shyly we smile at each other. His front teeth slightly overlap. And while I know it's probably irrational, I decide I love this small flaw and hope he never fixes it.

"Does your house look like this?" I ask him. I nod toward the tree.

"Well at Easter we usually have baskets with stuffed bunnies and my sisters dye eggs."

I laugh—but imagine his sisters running downstairs on Christmas morning in slippers and robes to rip open their presents. "They still believe in Santa Claus?"

"The two youngest."

I realize I want to believe in Santa Claus and the Easter Bunny. I want to believe in Tinkerbell. But I also want to believe in Jesus, God, or Zeus. It doesn't matter.

"You go to church for Christmas?"

"Christmas Eve."

I imagine the flame of white tapered candles reflecting on stained-glass windows. I imagine the scent of incense and the rustle of silk robes. I imagine voices singing Christmas hymns, imagine Christopher standing with his family, all in a row. When they return home after the service, his father will build a fire and his mother will fix hot chocolate. Christopher will plug in the tree, and his sisters will hold hands and whisper to each other what they hope Santa will bring them. And I want this as much as the church service, *this:* the fireplace, the hot chocolate, the lights on the tree. I imagine his sisters preparing for bed. I see them brushing their teeth and changing into pajamas. I see them pulling back sheets and nestling against pillows. But then, I don't know what else to see, what else I'm supposed to see. I want Christopher to tell me. Tell me: *How do your sisters sleep through night until morning? How much does your father love his daughters? What does he do to show it?*

When the next record begins to play, Christopher takes my hand and we dance. His skin is warm from the fire, and I see tiny licks of flame reflecting in his eyes. In the foyer just past the tree a few couples pretend to dance. It is dark there; they sway, don't dance. Boys run hands the length of girls' backs, pulling them closer. I think I can almost feel those hands on *my* back, on *my* shoulders. But no, stop—I don't want that. I don't want, could never want, that which happened with Steve, with Christopher. Surely I'm not even that girl anymore and no longer remember her name. With Christopher, I will never be that girl again. With Christopher, I am a shy suburban girl and surely no other. As I dance with him I feel drugged by his warmth, drugged by the scent of pine and cinnamon candles. But it is a gentle warmth. The skin on his hands is slightly rough. It is boy skin: skin that plays sports, skin that tinkers with engines. Safe skin. Skin too shy to touch girls' bodies.

Christopher's father waits in a red Rambler. We rush through the snow laughing, skidding. Christopher holds my hand. I hold on tight—my feet have missed years of practice walking on ice. Wind tingles my fire-warm cheeks, and I am breathless when we reach the car, breathless with cold and with this teenage girl giggle bubbling from my lips. Then, it is okay I don't have a Christmas tree, the myths, the hot chocolate. Now, at this moment, what I *do* have—flecks of snow on our eyelashes, his hand ensuring I don't slip—is enough. I have enough.

But I don't want it to stop. Rather, I want to stop time so this will last forever. The car moves slowly through unplowed streets, and my feet press the floorboards as if they're brakes, as if I can stop it. I want to think of something to say to Christopher's father to stop us. I want to spend the night in their home, in a sleeping bag on the floor of the room with his sisters. I want to be Christopher's sister. But we turn down Lowell Road, aiming toward my porch light.

Now, walking up the path, Christopher and I are not laughing. My grimness, which he will never, over the years, understand, which I will never be able to explain, is nevertheless contagious. I know this. Shyly we say good-night. There are thanks for a wonderful time, but as he turns to go I reach for his arm. He glances at me, questioning, slightly impatient. His father is watching, and I don't know how to explain why I have touched him, why I have stopped him, why I have called him back. I know no words to explain how badly I want him to save me. When I say nothing he gently tugs away.

And now he is returning to the car where his father waits, the engine running. I watch as he opens the car door, imagining the warmth of the heater. I wish he and his father would glance in the rearview mirror to see me, as if this glance could then carry me with them. I watch the taillights until they turn left on Rutland. There are no other cars on these streets. No other people. In small, silent furies, snowflakes whirl around globes of streetlights. I turn the knob on my front door, not wanting to touch this metal, instead wanting to remember the texture of Christopher's warm wool sweater.

□ □ □

I sit in the kitchen watching my mother peel potatoes for dinner. My father is not yet home, nor is my sister. My mother tells me stories from her childhood, about growing up in Chicago during the

Depression. Her father taught himself English by reading the dictionary. Uncles, aunts, cousins were always passing through, dropping in for breakfast or dinner. They slept two, sometimes three, to a bed.

"What about your father?" I ask.

For a moment she stops peeling and looks at me. She shrugs. She tells me he was a Socialist, that he cared about the Workers, that he didn't have time for his five children, barely had time to earn a living. He was always at meetings, but they were happier when he was gone, she says, laughing, because he had a terrible temper.

She tells me: They didn't have enough money for food. One day her mother walked down the street to borrow an egg from a neighbor and on her way home she dropped it. She retrieved it in a saucer and still used it.

She tells me: We never had enough to eat. We were always hungry.

She tells me: We're lucky your father earns a good living. You don't know what it feels like to go to bed hungry.

She tells me: Things aren't always the way you want them, but you have to manage. That's what I learned to do. Get by. Manage.

She tells me: No one has a happy childhood. Everyone's got problems.

I hear the garage door open. My father is home. I stand and begin to walk down the hall toward my bedroom. "Yes, Mom," I say. "But just because you have enough food doesn't mean you can't still go to bed hungry."

□ □ □

What I don't notice in novels: that the fathers in the novels don't touch their daughters the way mine touches me. Yet while I don't believe our relationship strange, I would never tell anyone about it. These contradictions are logical. Contradictions are always logical. Now, even though our family lacks a Christmas tree, still I believe we are exceedingly normal.

□ □ □

This year I receive Christmas cards even before I mail mine. Again I decorate my room with them, but no longer is this enough. After Robin's party, I must have a tree. I ask my parents if we can get one, just this once. No angels or religious ornaments, just a tree. "No." If I don't spend money on decorations? Our presents would look so pretty under a tree. "No." I'll use my own allowance. I'll make all the decorations myself. We'll put it in some corner where it'll hardly show, where no one would see it. "No."

Every day I walk to the lot next to the railroad tracks where trees are sold, watch fathers lift trees atop cars and tie them securely. Mothers slide trees into the backs of station wagons. In the evening, after the last commuter train pulls from the small station, the man who owns the trees leaves, without locking the lot. I head toward home, slamming my boots in puddles of melted snow. It is past dusk, and green, red, white outdoor Christmas lights glitter on eaves and doors and windows. On one house a giant Santa is attached to a chimney. Magical blue lights twinkle on every tree and bush in another yard. Ours is the only house on Lowell Road without magic, without lights.

Two days before Christmas, when I get off the bus from Ridgewood where I'd gone to buy presents, I notice the price of trees has been cut in half. The owner wears a blue ski cap pulled low on his forehead, and he sits on a wood crate smoking a cigarette. I wonder if he's noticed me standing in this same spot every day. I don't care. I set the shopping bag by my feet and watch the few remaining trees that haven't been purchased. Most of them are scraggly, with branches broken or missing. Even with the price cut, the man sells few trees. Today I abandon my vigil before he closes, lugging home my shopping bag of Christmas presents.

My Christmas presents. In Ridgewood, all the stores had smelled of tinsel and golden perfume. I had bought my sister a book, my mother a wool scarf, my father a necktie. These presents are unoriginal, but it doesn't matter. Kiki will thank me profusely for the book she will never read. My mother will inspect the scarf as if it has moth holes. My father will adore his necktie, wear it every day, but never truly see it: I could have bought a tie with any design, in any color.

On Christmas Eve my sister is home early since all her friends are with their families. She is upstairs in her room, the door shut. I am downstairs in my room, the door shut. A symphony blares on the record player in the living room, the walls of the house shuddering in sound. For hours my father will play his music, even though we, his three little girls, detest it. Still, we would not consider asking him to lower the volume.

My mother is in her bedroom, *their* bedroom, her door also shut to avoid the music. But I want my mother to be in the kitchen. There are no scents of special foods. There are no Christmas cookies or cakes. Not a shred of a decoration or sign of Christmas joy. Although they couldn't possibly be, my feet feel frozen, and I sit on my bed holding them, trying to warm them, believing they are iced solid enough to kick my mother's bedroom door to pieces, kick my father's record player into the street.

For dinner my mother serves hamburgers and potato chips. This emphatic gesture is her response to Christmas, since she believes it a personal affront to her Jewishness. While every family across the Christian world decorates trees, cooks special foods, buys presents, and prays in churches, my mother will believe each decoration, each cookie, each present, each prayer, is an attempt to rob her of her self. There is no room in her heart for those who are different. My father imagines himself more generous. He believes he is a great humanitarian who loves everyone.

I drench the burger in ketchup before devouring it, barely chewing, barely tasting meat, swallowing chunks in order to appease my ravenous hunger. My fingers are sticky with ketchup but I don't stop to wipe them, nor can I stop eating chips. My mother has bought only one bag. I eat most of it, and my sister is angry. I eat a plain bun, without a hamburger, soaking it in ketchup until it is soggy. I eat four dill pickles, but it is bread I need, starch, or meat, foods far more solid than pickles. I suck my fingers. I need more food, more potato chips, more something. I press a damp finger to the bottom of the bag for the remaining crumbs of chips. Even salt. I suck my fingers for the last grain. Still, I need more . . . more meat, more starch, more salt. I need more now. So without plan, not caring that stores are closed, in fact not even considering this, I yank on my jacket. My parents yell at me: Where are you going? I don't know. It doesn't matter. I must go, go, go. They can't stop me. Threats are useless. What could they possibly threaten to do? I can't stop moving.

The wind seems to propel me toward town. This is how quickly I seem to be walking. Snowy puddles have iced—I have forgotten my boots—and I skid on leather-soled shoes, without slipping or falling, skid as if the ice itself is part of this plan to hurry me along. I am not in my mind; rather, it is my slick feet which understand the destination. I do not. Nothing could stop them; nothing could even try. But maybe it *is* my mind urging my feet forward, a mind suddenly galvanized, now clearly focused, free of the bounds of home.

Surely I know I have not come to town for potato chips that would not be for sale tonight anyway. Instead, I am at the Christmas tree lot where the owner is long gone. Lights from the train station reveal the few trees leaning against a makeshift wire fence. Easy access. No gate, no lock. No one to say no. The streets are deserted. No witnesses. Never have I been so close. Now, finally, I will enter the lot, this for the first time.

Most of the trees have broken branches. Dented sides. Crushed needles. Some are too thin, some too short and stumpy. This doesn't matter. Although I know I will take one, what I want, for the moment, is just to be with the trees. All of them. How can I choose just one? I have forgotten my mittens and I move closer to them, my arms outstretched, until the tips of my fingers can almost smell dark-scented pine. I move deep into their midst until I am surrounded by them, hidden by them, believe I could almost *be* one of them.

But these trees shouldn't have to be hidden in this lot without Christmas lights. I trail a finger along the wire fence until it vibrates in friction, warming it, warming my finger, until the wire is humming in a blaze of flashing lights. The lot shimmers. The trees seem decorated in glitter. Wands of light beam out to the stars; the stars echo back, drizzling stardust onto the gentlest green branches. Thousands of birds shed white feathers to dust the pine needles with snow. Rings from Saturn encircle the treetops with halos. Icy diamonds stud the boughs.

And now I don't search for the best tree but rather the worst: the tree no one would ever buy. Not out of guilt over the steal—hardly. Rather, I want it. This one tree. Walking backward, I drag it home by the base. The journey seems to take hours. My arms ache. My shoulder blades cramp. The bark scratches my hands, but when I pause to rest and press my palms to my face, I smell dark, rich sap. It warms me. I continue on, dizzy in the backward movement, in my abrupt steps. The wind gusts my hair around my face, but I don't let go of the tree to brush it aside. Up the path to my house, up the steps to the front stoop, I pull it. As I push the tree inside, the storm door slams against it. No one comes to inquire about the noise. Certainly no one would help me. I lug the tree across the living room carpet and down the hall to my bedroom.

I have no stand in which to place the tree, so I lean it against the wall and secure it with every book in my shelf. I pop popcorn and string it, draping it round and round. With construction paper, I glue together circles of red, green, purple, and gold and loop the chain from the top of the tree to the bottom. I hang garlands of aluminum foil crunched to glittering balls. I thread my Christmas cards and dangle them from branches. Dabs of Pepsodent toothpaste are flecks of snow. From every brush in the bathroom I comb out the hairs. I brush my own hair a hundred times, pull the strands from the brush, then brush it another hundred. I mat and mold all the hair into a bird nest and balance it atop the tree. Small wads of white paper are eggs, and I cut a dove from a piece of gray paper. With crayons, I draw the crèche I'd seen at Robin's and wrap it around the base. In my darkened room I prop a flashlight on the floor and beam it up through the branches. I smell the sap, the popcorn, the peace. Tonight no one comes near the door to my room; tonight no one would dare invade this alien room of peaceful Christmas spirits.

The next morning, Christmas day, my parents and my sister enter my room to see my earth-green shrine. I believe they think it pretty, although they say little. That afternoon my father builds a fire in the fireplace. I sit on the couch and feel warmth flare about the room. On the coffee table is a monkeypod bowl filled with oranges and walnuts. Snips of flame reflect in the silver nutcracker. The record player is not turned on, nor is the radio. Our house is quiet. I breathe quietly, listening to the click of needles as my mother knits me a sweater. My sister sits next to me, turning the pages of the book I bought her for Christmas.

□ □ □

Christopher invites me to the following dances: Harbor Lights, Paradise of Hearts, Hawaiian Dream. I buy new dresses, cut my hair again, select lipsticks to match my new clothes. We attend parties together. We walk together in the halls between classes. We exchange pictures. Finally, he holds my hand. My parents have no objections to him—how could they? He is a shy, sweet boy. Except sometimes, when he and I are dancing, I glance away from this shy, sweet boy and watch Ryan, who dances with both arms encircling a girl. I think I can feel the taut muscles in his arms as he presses her to him, his eyes closed. The girl holds him, too, her face cradled between his neck and his shoulder. Sometimes I want Christopher like this. I want Christopher to hold me tight and stroke me. Otherwise, how can I know he loves me? But do I really want this? Maybe I want Christopher the way he is. It is that girl, the one with long blonde hair, the one who desires my father and Ryan—*she* is the one who wants Christopher to be like Ryan. Truly, I could belong to Christopher or to Ryan. If I belong to someone else, then I can't be alone with my self.

□ □ □

Elizabeth invites me to her pajama party. I take this literally–that I must bring pajamas. But my mother won't give me money to buy pajamas; she says what I sleep in—that nightgown—is what I will bring . . . she will not waste money on . . . on what? Suddenly I am not sure about any of my clothes. Once I wore a tight knit sweater to school and I thought I noticed a surprised hesitation to Christopher's "hello." At the time I thought little of it, but now I'm unsure. My mother helped me select the ruby-red dress I wore to the Paradise of Hearts dance. The cut was lower than the cut on other girls' dresses. But my mother says it's okay to look this way—it's important to attract boys, just don't allow them to touch you.

While I stood before the full-length mirror examining myself in that red dress, my mother came up behind me and cupped her hands over my breasts. She told me I was developing nicely. But I don't understand. I don't understand this body. Why do I think my father hates these breasts that are developing, hates this hair growing on my body—breasts and hair that seem to be beyond his or my control? Why do I think he wants me to remain his little girl—always? I don't know how my body should look. I don't know what kind of body would make my mother and father happy—would make Christopher happy. Must I have three bodies, and three sets of clothes, in order to keep everyone happy? Or if I discover the right clothes, will I then have the right body?

So when I receive the invitation to the pajama party, I'm scared all my clothes are wrong: for school, for dances, for pajama parties—wrong for Christopher. I take the bus to Ridgewood and wander the aisles at Sealfons, where my friends shop, usually not where my mother and I buy clothes. Blue, pink, and white Oxford shirts with button-down collars. Plaid sweater-and-skirt sets, loose fitting, with matching kneesocks. Well, yes, I have clothes like these, too, but Sealfons sells no ruby-red dresses or tight knit sweaters. I know I am wrong, wrong, wrong. The clothes here are teenage clothes, while my mother takes me to stores for adults. And I know I cannot bring a nightgown to Elizabeth's party.

I wander to the sleepware section and study exotic flannel pajamas. Pink. Yellow. Blue. I take a blue pair with white flowers into the dressing room, slip off my skirt and sweater, and try them on. Perfect. They fit loosely, showing no contours of my body. I smooth my hands over the fabric. I believe if I owned these I would be able to curl inside them and sleep undisturbed for years, smelling and feeling their warm comfort. I have no money, but I must own these pajamas. I must steal them—I *must*. I cannot leave without them. I roll the cuffs to my knees, put my skirt on, pull my sweater over the top, and zip up my jacket. Slowly, I leave the store.

Since I want the pajamas to remain new and clean and pretty, the way I know the other girls' pajamas will be, I wait for the night of the party to wear them. Once I shed my school clothes, button the top of the pajamas, and slip my legs into the bottoms, I safely blend into the group of girls. Camouflaged in my flannel uniform, I smile, pleased I made the right choice, all by myself, on what to wear for the party.

Our sleeping bags, blankets, and pillows are spread across the carpeted living room floor. Our overnight cases spill scarves, underwear, socks. We roll each other's hair in plastic rollers. We paint each other's fingernails with pink and white pearly polish. We paint our toenails, too, stuffing cotton between our toes as described in *Seventeen*. We play rock 'n' roll records and dance—alone and with each other. We eat bags of chips and drink bottles of pop. At midnight, Elizabeth's mother brings us boxes of doughnuts: jelly, cinnamon, cream. We laugh. We gossip about boys and tell secrets. "You think Christopher'll ask you to go steady?" Robin asks me.

"I don't know," I say. "Maybe. I hope so."

"My mom says I'm too young to 'get involved,'" Elizabeth says.

Quickly I glance down at my pink nails, worried I might have given the wrong answer. "Oh, of course," I say. "My mom tells me the same thing."

"It's not like you gotta do everything your mother tells you," Robin says. She tells us her mom allows her to kiss her boyfriend only if she keeps her feet on the floor. Except she demonstrates how it's possible to *lie* on a couch and still keep at least one foot on the floor. We all practice. I am slow to learn this; I am, I must be, the most innocent of all.

Late at night I go to the bathroom. I drift down the hall away from the girls still playing records, still talking. The door to the bathroom is closed, so I wait, admiring my new pajamas. I press the crook of my arm to my face, breathing the material. It smells good and new. And suddenly I am afraid to sleep in them, afraid when I wake in the morning they will no longer smell clean or good or new. Perhaps I should slip them off while everyone is sleeping and change into my clothes.

The door opens and I pull back, surprised. I'd assumed one of the girls was inside, but it's Elizabeth's father in his robe. He holds the door open, but I can't move—I don't understand—I'm confused by his sudden presence in this nighttime hall. He smiles and jokes—I barely hear him—something about girls and noise and fun. I mean, what he says is *nice*. His smile is nice. That's all it is, but I can't respond. I fear my new pajamas will be criticized. He will tell me to change them. No, he will unbutton them. He will . . . but he doesn't do any of this. He walks down the hall to a bedroom. He opens a door. As he does I hear a woman, his wife, say something to him. From the tone, what she says doesn't seem to be significant, probably: "Please, turn off the light." She is not angry. Nor is she silent. The door closes. For a moment there is a rim of light beneath the door, but then it disappears. The room he shares with his wife is dark. Still I can't move. I lean against the wall and close my eyes. I think I am waiting for something. I wait for that door to open again. He will return, come back down the hall, silently. No one will hear. Except everyone hears. But he does it anyway because he can't stop.

But that door—the door behind which Elizabeth's father sleeps with his wife—does not open. He does not walk back down the hall. How do I know he sleeps in that room all night? How do I know he doesn't leave it? Maybe from the definite way the door tapped shut. Maybe from the sound of his wife's voice. Maybe from the still air here in the hall, air that will not be disturbed again until morning. Or maybe because I believe Elizabeth's mother knows how to teach her daughter, knows how to guide her.

For the briefest of moments—more a sense than one clear thought—I understand that what I do every night is not repeated in every other girl's bedroom, down every street and block, in every neighborhood, all across town. Had I believed that what I do with my father is usual? I don't know, I don't know, I don't know. But then, as definitively as Elizabeth's father shut the door to the bedroom he shares with his wife, that thought—the thought that I might be alone, that what I do is not repeated, is not normal—is slammed from my mind.

All night I'm awake. I'm afraid someone will see me if I change into my clothes, so I lie awake in my pajamas, not moving, not wanting to wrinkle them. I spread my arms to the sides so I won't sweat on the clean material. I think I know my love for these pajamas is irrational—at least I know the other girls don't seem concerned about theirs—but I want these pajamas to last the rest of my life. They have to. But I'm scared they will be taken from me. They will be ripped; they will be ruined. That place between my legs feels safe behind the tightly sewn seam. But I have this small dread the seam might split. So I don't move my legs. I lie perfectly still until morning.

On Monday I neatly refold the pajamas along the creases, smooth the material, and return the pajamas to the store, leaving them in a paper bag in the dressing room. I must. I would not be able to bear seeing the pajamas wrinkled.

□ □ □

Next week is Posture Week in junior high and each grade will award medals for Posture King and Queen. So badly do I need this medal, I can't even think of a reason why. Maybe because I've never before won an award. Maybe I imagine myself proudly announcing my award to my parents one night at dinner. Maybe because I know I'll never win an award for academics. But the reason doesn't matter. I simply must win, must be Posture Queen for Ninth Grade. Over the weekend I practice walking with a book on my head. I stand with my back flat against the wall until my shoulders hurt. I sit on the edge of my bed ramrod straight until the muscles in my back ache. Then I force myself to sit like that even longer. My image of good posture has little to do with grace. It has to do with rigidity, inflexibility, stiffness. It has to do with a body immobilized and mute.

During each class period the teacher observes the students and hands out a wood chip to the one displaying the best posture. At the end of the day each student turns in his or her chips to the homeroom teacher, and at the end of the week the chips are tallied and the student with the most wins. I do little during class except sit rigid. I can't take notes because I'd have to bend over the desk to write. My hands are neatly folded on top of the desk. My feet are flat on the floor. My neck is stiff, my gaze forward, my shoulders back. I can control my body. At the end of the first day, I have four chips.

By Thursday my back is so sore it hurts to walk, but I would never consider abandoning my goal. At the end of English, the teacher forgets to hand out chips and I know I can't depart without one. I linger, hover by her desk, ask a question about the homework assignment—while watching the wood chips stacked next to her box of pencils. I must have one. If she turns her head I might steal one—or all of them. After she answers my question, I continue to stand rigidly by her desk. I'm not leaving. I try to will her to remember the chips, will her to give one to me, but she doesn't understand why I linger.

"Those chips—" I nod toward them but am afraid to actually ask for one.

She glances at them. "Oh—I forgot to hand them out," she says.

"I've been practicing my posture," I say.

She glances at my empty desk as if I still sit there and she can see me. "Yes," she says. "I think I remember your posture." She picks up a wood chip. "Would you like one?"

I grab it from her hand before it's fully offered. "Can I have two?" I say. "I know I'll have just as good posture tomorrow."

At assembly on Friday my name is announced: Posture Queen of the Ninth Grade. I'm called to the stage while everyone applauds. I am enormously proud as I receive a small silver medal. Walking home, I hold it in my palm. I realize the possibility that no one else even tried to win this, but I don't care. I decide I'll wait till dinner to announce my award to my parents. At home I lie on my bed and try to relax my muscles, the first time all week. Over and over I read the inscription: "Posture Queen—Ninth Grade." I'm sorry my name's not on it, but of course there wasn't time to engrave it. I place the medal on my forehead as if it's a gem for an exotic religious ritual—that Egyptian princess. Then I place it first over my left eye, then the right. With my eyes closed I concentrate on the cool weighted circle over my eye. It feels like a mark. Like the cross drawn on my forehead on Good Friday at the Anglican school in St. Thomas. My body is special. My body, my posture, have been selected, elected, anointed.

All through dinner the medal remains on my lap as I wait for a good time for my announcement. But then I can't. I can't say it. Why? Certainly my father will praise it. My mother will wave its smallness aside. My sister will refuse to look at it. I already know their responses—but, really, this isn't why I can't tell them. Now I realize I must keep it secret. While my body is special, *no one can know this secret. This* is why I had to win the medal. My body needed to receive its special mark. But as I leave the table and return to my room, the glory is fading. I need to be able to win it all over again next week as well.

□ □ □

I graduate from junior high school. The previous summer I saw none of my friends. This summer I am included in the promise we'll all meet at the swimming pool. At home I try on the bathing suit I bought last summer but never wore. Immediately I see it's too small and ask my mother if I can buy a new one. She refuses, since this one is "just like new." Besides, we see the suit differently.

My mother says it fits, and that's that. But my breasts, I think, are not sufficiently hidden behind the material. Before my first trip to the pool I stand before the bathroom mirror, trying to arrange the top of the suit. I loosen the straps. I tighten them. I put on a shirt and tie the shirttails together across my stomach. I roll the sleeves up. Maybe I'll just take the shirt off at the last moment, before I enter the water.

I grab a towel. As I head toward the door my father comes in from the yard where he's building a brick patio. His hands are dirty, and he calls to me from the kitchen to pour him a glass of ice water. I give it to him, but he sets it down and holds onto my hand instead. I'm not wearing shorts over the suit, only the shirt, and I lower the towel to cover my thighs. He tugs it away and asks where I'm going, dressed like that. To the pool, I say. I'm supposed to meet my friends. I'm already late, I add. He says he needs my help with the patio. Can I help later? I ask. I'll work on it all day tomorrow, Sunday. He reminds me he and my mother have an engagement tomorrow. He won't be working on it then. He needs me now. He needs me today. But I'm already in my bathing suit, I say . . .

I should stop this. I know it. I feel his anger; he wears it tight on the skin round his mouth. He tells me to change, unbuttons my shirt and—there is the bathing suit, too small, yes. Now I see it clearly. I see I could not possibly go to the pool anyway. Not in this suit. The shirt is on the floor and his anger, rising: You will never go to the pool in that suit, he says, and I nod, yes, yes, of course, this is all a mistake. I had planned not to swim, not to remove the shirt anyway, I whisper. One of the straps is in his hand and he jerks it so hard it snaps. The top of the suit slips, and my breast—there. I don't know where my mother is. I think I hear her in the living room, just past the door of the kitchen. He speaks to me, but

I have trouble concentrating, trouble connecting words to their meaning. He asks if I'd expected to go to the pool like this? No, I shake my head, no. Really, this is a mistake, I say. I don't know what I'd been thinking. I wasn't going. I wasn't. I won't. I'll help you with the patio, Father. I try to cover my breast with my hand, but he hits it.

With the sound, my mother is there in the kitchen and I'm afraid to try to cover my breast again, cover its overwhelming embarrassment. They are yelling at each other. I don't understand what I have done. What they have done. What any of us have done. She says I'm his slutdaughter, and that's how I'll always dress. And he says, what, like her? Didn't she dress like a slut before they married?

And there her rage is, all her rage, screaming at him. Her face is unbearable. She is almost laughing, too, I think, gleeful that somehow she has tricked him, but I don't understand how, or what the trick has been. There is glee, too, that he will not be the only one to control my body, that, yes, he has been doubly tricked. And how about *him*, she says, doesn't she know what he, my father, did with his own whore mother? And hasn't she always known their secret?

At the mention of his mother I feel his rage darken, and he picks up a knife and for a moment just grips it. There is so much rage, hers and his, the soles of my feet feel the floorboards shudder. He walks toward her with the knife, but she is laughing at him now, just laughing, high and strained, and she takes her purse from the counter and heads to the garage. The sound of his breathing seems louder than the engine of the car starting. He steps toward me but I know it is not me, his daughter, he sees standing before him, but surely another, some ancient, ancient image. He slices the other strap of her suit, nicking her. He grabs her hair, the hair belonging to that other, pulling her to the floor. Pulls off her suit. The knife—he puts the knife there, between her legs there. But surely his slutdaughter deserves this. Yes, I see what he does to his slutdaughter, before her body turns to granite. I feel nothing. There is nothing to feel. Perhaps splinters of granite chip from her skin as I see him cut her there, moments before he fucks her.

We are on the kitchen floor. I don't remember time, but long enough for his rage to chip, chip at the granite, yet barely leave a scar. The granite is hard enough, thick enough, to last his rage a lifetime. *I will help you, Daddy, help you cauterize your rage.* I know that I must. I know this is why I was born, this is why I am here. I know he feels better after, and only I can help him with this. He must love me more than he loves my mother, more than he loves my sister. I am the one to coax his rage from his body, urging it from his body deep into mine.

In the late afternoon the sky is still pale, flecked with silvery light of early summer. I follow my father outside, since he wants us to work on the patio together. From the mound of sand in the driveway we load smaller piles into the wheelbarrow and roll it to the back door where the patio is to be. The sand is the bed. With rakes, we smooth it across the sectioned-off earth before placing green and gray bricks on top. Four-inch strips of white pebbles will separate the rows. While we work we don't speak, except when he tells me how to arrange pebbles, how to rake sand. By the time fireflies decorate the sky, we're only half finished. He says we'll finish on Monday.

Inside, he places cream cheese, pumpernickel bread, a bowl of cherries and grapes on the kitchen counter. He places two plates in front of us, where we stand side by side. He is ravenous, eating quickly, and I think if I watch his mouth chew I will vomit. I pick up a grape. Between my fingers it feels slick and pulpy, and I feel vomit begin to rise. The base of my throat is hot and tight. I must get out of the kitchen.

Without a word I go down the hall to the bathroom and stand over the sink, turning both faucets until water gushes. I don't even touch the water, just watch it swirl into the pink bowl and down the drain. I am sweaty. My hair is matted. My whole body needs washing. I can't take a shower. I'm afraid to feel water on my skin. I don't want to feel this. I'm afraid the granite will dissolve—but it can't, I tell myself. Granite can't feel. Can't. Never have I touched that one place on my body that's never been identified by word—only identified by need, by what he needs. Sometimes I quickly slide a bar of soap over it, sometimes a washcloth. Never have I looked at myself. I don't want to see, don't want to know. But it needs washing. I need washing. I wet my hands and press them to my cheeks, but there it is, *there,* I must stop, for with the wetness against my cheeks the skin *does* feel. It feels softer. I can't do this.

My father comes in the bathroom and asks what I'm doing. I can't answer him; I don't know what I'm doing. He turns off the faucets and stands behind me, stroking my hair. I want him to see it's matted, that it needs to be washed and brushed. He doesn't see this, would never notice this. I must tell him: "My hair is dirty, Daddy."

He looks at me, surprised. "Your hair is beautiful. You have the most beautiful hair in the world."

"It needs to be *washed,* Daddy." My voice hits hard against the tiles in the bathroom.

"That's okay, then," he says. He touches my shoulder, trying to lower my voice. "It's okay to wash it."

"But I need to be cleaned." I am almost crying. "Daddy. I don't know how to do it."

"You're my precious," he says. "Whatever you want. I'll clean you."

He doesn't understand what I'm saying; I don't understand how to explain.

While the bathtub fills we sit beside each other on the edge. Now, for this moment, he seems tired. He holds his bent head in his hand, his eyes closed. He doesn't notice the water near the top. I am the one to turn it off and slide into the tub. Then he looks at me and wets the bar of soap to wash me. I begin to feel myself disperse. I am the steam. Each molecule of my body vaporizes into transparent beads of mist. He soaps his hand and washes, washes this body, but doesn't he know he touches nothing?

"You're my most precious girl," he says to me. His hand is there, between my legs. "Tell me," he whispers. "I know. Tell me how much you want it again. Tell me how much you love it."

He always says this to me, says he knows when I want him, when my body wants him, and only him. But I don't understand what it is he feels there, how it is he can tell. And I don't understand how he can say this, now when I hurt, when I couldn't possibly want anything. So I can't—I can't tell him the only words he ever wants to hear me say. Instead, I pull away from him slightly, knowing I shouldn't, knowing this will make him angry, make him want it more.

The movement had been slight, but he notices. His fingers are rigid, ordering me not to move. He tells me to unzip his shorts, tells me to make him the way I love him. And I want to say to him: *Daddy, no, no. What we need now is sleep.* I say nothing. He won't see, will never see, our exhaustion. I know our bodies are finite. He's too quickly using them up.

So Celeste smiles. Evil. Disdainful. Taunting. This slutdaughter. Her smile shows short evil teeth as she reaches for his penis.

His hand guides hers, but she can't get it right tonight, can't get him hard enough. They're too tired. He won't listen to his exhaustion. His tension is greater, and he squeezes her hand tight around it. He makes her move faster, tries to get her hand to grip it tighter, and she's focused on it, but she can't do it, can't do it right, and he's angry now. He yanks her shoulder up until she's kneeling and he says for her to suck it. He holds her by the throat to guide her mouth to the proper rhythm but she can't do this right either, and when she begins to gag, her taunting smile is far away and she is pulled from the tub and is on the floor, water streaming from her body. He has to have an orgasm. She knows this. He has to have one now. It is the most important thing in her life, to give him one. She knows that once he's this far, there is no way to stop or go back, that she must do everything she can to draw it from his body. He is angry. He smears petroleum jelly on her and touches her where she's sore, his fingers hurting her, hurting inside her, there—and when she begins to kick at him to stop he rubs her harder until she pleads with him and then, finally, when she is weeping—he loves to see her weep—he is hard now, strong, ready to fuck her. And he does.

Sunday morning, I stay in my bedroom until I hear my parents leave the house. Then I go into the bathroom. No one has bothered to drain the bathtub from last night. Quickly I flip the lever and thoroughly rinse the gritty residue at the bottom with cleanser and a sponge. I wash my face and brush my teeth. My hair is still dirty and tangled. I drag the brush through it, unraveling snarls. I lean over the sink and splash water on my hair until it is damp. I part it, making sure the part is as straight as possible.

In the kitchen, I wipe the counter and put the dishes from the night before in the dishwasher. I spread peanut butter on a slice of bread and stand by the window. The unfinished patio and yard are in disarray with clods of earth, mounds of sand, scattered bricks, rakes, shovels. I don't want the outside of our house to be messy. I don't want to see the patio unfinished, looking hastily abandoned. I'm sure my parents hate for our yard to be this way, too. How pleased they would be to return home to a house with a beautiful new patio. They would love me so much if I am the one to suddenly conjure it for them, like magic. I pull on shorts, a shirt, sneakers and go outside.

All day I load sand and bricks in the wheelbarrow and cart them to the patio. I arrange each brick carefully in the sand, each brick in the perfectly symmetrical design, each row separated by four inches of white pebbles. At dusk I turn on the outside spotlights and continue, row by row. The skin on my hands is scratched, my muscles ache, but I barely notice. I have to finish the patio. I feel enormous gratification at the neatness, the orderliness, of each row.

Soon after ten my parents turn into the drive. I rush to meet the car before they pull into the garage. I open the doors and urge them to hurry, come with me, see what I've done. Proudly, I display the patio and walk across each row of bricks, needing to demonstrate how solidly the bricks are settled. My parents are amazed I finished it by myself. Yes, I say. All by myself. I did this for you. I am beaming. They come to me and hug me, admiring it, testing it themselves, exclaiming what a fine job I've done. "It adds so much to the house," they say. Yes, the house. Our house must look perfect, like Jane's house, like Christopher's house, perfect for everyone to admire.

We are that New Jersey family, then, admiring our New Jersey house. It is brick with dark gray trim surrounded by a mowed lawn and weeded flower beds. We are that family—we are you, any of you, up and down Lowell Road, standing in our nighttime yard with the spotlight arcing across our newly completed patio. We are that family in the photograph—the one snapped, for example, at the opening of my father's bank in Saddle Brook. We three girls wear white gloves, nylon stockings, wool suits. My mother and my sister wear dark velvet hats. A white hair-band secures my hair. My father, in a suit, has an arm around me, where he stands between my mother and me, proudly. My sister always stands slightly detached from the family, but no one would consider this curious. Not in that photograph. Nor would anyone notice anything curious in this one, where we stand together admiring our house and our yard.

Because we can be that family, too—*this* family. Families don't exist in one dimension only. Who was my family last night? Last night we had centuries of civilization stripped from our skin. Last night we devolved through centuries of time, to a beach white as salt, and as dry. But tonight, as we admire our patio, we're just like you and like you, we can *be* you, when we really, really try.

□ □ □

A month has passed since my father ripped the straps of my bathing suit. Finally, one Monday morning when he is at the bank and my mother is shopping, I decide to repair them. I sit on my bed with my mother's sewing box. I double the thread for strength. This will hold, as I've already decided I won't actually go swimming. And no one will see the stitches, since I'll wear a shirt over the suit, as before.

By noon I head toward the pool. I haven't seen anyone all summer, and I'm scared I won't be accepted. Scared my friends won't invite me to put my towel beside them. Scared I'll be ignored.

Scared there are marks on my body that everyone will notice. Just this morning I shaved my legs to the knee. The skin feels overexposed, my bare legs awkward, walking outside on the street. Heat from the pavement softens the soles of my white Ked sneakers and seems to reflect too brightly off the surface of my calves and thighs. I'm scared of what someone might see.

My friends sit on the grass outside the chain-link fence surrounding the pool. I grip my towel to my chest and slowly walk toward them. A transistor radio plays. Skin gleams with suntan lotion. Many have summer tans. Relief: I am not told to go elsewhere. Everyone invites me to place my towel here, or here—you'll get better sun here. Where've you been all summer? I say I had to help my father build a patio. This is accepted. Yet the girls in the group are nervous, I can tell, and I wonder what's wrong. As I sit beside Robin she touches my hand, asking my eyes to follow her gaze down the length of the grass to a smaller group of kids from school. Christopher. He's with a girl named Lynn. Robin whispers she's seen them together from the beginning of summer. No one knows how he could possibly like her more than me—but then Lynn is not part of our crowd.

I pretend I'm not upset, yet all I want to do is run back to my home, to my room. I can't speak. For a moment all I do is watch Christopher. If I stare long enough, maybe the forcefulness of my gaze will erase him. Robin advises me to forget him, pretend I'm interested in another guy. She whispers that Ryan broke up with his girlfriend and lists other available guys. "We're all going to Palisades Park on Saturday and we won't invite Christopher," she says. "He'll see. He'll regret it. Ask one of the guys to go swimming."

One of the guys. Ryan lies on a towel at the edge of the group, reading. The tips of his fingers carelessly flick pages of a magazine.

He drums them against paper as he pauses to glance at a picture. What I'd felt in Steve's fingers I now feel in Ryan's—that urgency, that need. I lie back on my towel with the sun hot on my face, thinking of Ryan. With Ryan, I could be the girl who sneaks away from dances to have her back pushed against walls, her stomach hard against his. Now I understand I have worn this suit for Ryan, as if I knew all along I would be with him today, not with Christopher. With Christopher I would hide beneath my shirt, careful not to scare him. I know my body scares him. I know Ryan will never be scared. He will desire my body. The shyness I feel with Christopher is absent with Ryan. I will be much happier with Ryan.

She will be.

Celeste's blonde hair tumbles down my back. Her red lips pout in a smile as she sheds the shirt and leads Ryan into the swimming pool. She laughs and splashes him with water and dares him to jump off the high dive. He does. She watches, holding onto the side of the pool until he returns, shaking water from his eyes. Her arm drifts against his; their bodies drift in the movement of water, brushing against each other. When he turns to ask her something, his gaze lingers at the top of this too-small bathing suit. And Celeste smiles at him with her taunting eyes.

But I am the one who now notices Christopher and Lynn wade into the water. He says something and she laughs—her smile, *hers*, as shy as his. He holds her hand in a way he never held mine, because he *can* hold hers. Her hand doesn't threaten. And suddenly I understand why I'm not with Christopher. He knows about Celeste. Even though he has never seen me in this bathing suit, he knows about it—understands what it means. Like that tight knit sweater. He knows about . . . I don't let myself fully understand what he knows, but I believe that if he glances in my direction he will be horrified by what he sees.

I release the ledge and push myself far below water, straining against its bouyancy, kicking and cupping my hands to carry me down. Vibrations from swimmers rock against me. I feel a dull pounding in my ears, louder as I sink toward the bottom. I want to hear this pounding, nothing else. Chlorine burns my eyes, but I keep them open, wanting them burned. I know—I *know* what I will do with Ryan, and I know I will always miss Christopher, will always want him back. But I know I have done something too awful to deserve him—that I would have to be cleansed in order to get him back. All the water and astringents my mother pours into my body will not be enough. My body overwhelms me with disgust. I believe only if I drain all the blood from it will this horror that lives in it be gone.

Ryan swims to the bottom of the pool to find me, to pull me back up. I let him, let his hand brush the top of my suit, let his legs brush my thigh. When I reach the surface I am crying—it is only tears—I make no sound—and Ryan thinks my eyes are irritated from chlorine. He jokes: "I can make you feel better." I tell him, yes, I believe him. I know that he can.

At home I pull on slacks, a heavy shirt, socks. I put two blankets on the bed and huddle beneath them, shivering. My hair is damp, but I don't want to roll it or sit under the dryer. I press my hands between my knees, trying to warm them. I've closed windows and curtains to shut out light. I tell my mother I'm too sick to eat dinner. Later, she brings me a bowl of soup and Ritz crackers, my favorite, but when I pick up a cracker I begin to cry. She feels my forehead and says I'm warm and must take my temperature. I plead with her—no. At school the nurse uses a mouth thermometer, but we don't have that kind. I *can't* have my temperature taken, I tell her. I can't. I think I will scream if she takes it. She says if I'm not sick I have to eat, and if I'm sick she has to take my temperature and call the doctor.

My father comes in the room to see what's wrong. My mother pulls down the blankets, my slacks, my underwear. By now I am frigid with shame, and she's unable to insert the thermometer. They say I am stubborn and willful and that if I won't let them a doctor will make me. My mother slaps my thighs, but the cold deepens. I'm not breathing and feel as if I'm sinking back down in the water. I shiver harder. Only their anger is colder and harder than I, and I know I should not be doing this. They are right: I am a stubborn and willful child. To stop this, all I must do is let go. I must leave me, let who I am go, but I can't. I can't stop shivering.

My father tells my mother he will do it. He knows exactly where I keep the White Rose Petroleum Jelly and dabs some on the thermometer. But as I feel it enter I push back with a force, with an explosive strength I know is greater than I could ever be. I do not want my temperature taken. I fall over onto the mattress before sliding onto the floor. The thermometer breaks. I want this, yes. I am grateful.

I have slept. Or fainted. When I awake I'm on my bed with a doctor bending over me. Even with my eyes closed, I know my mother is in the room watching me, fascinated by what the doctor does to my body. To me, it doesn't matter what he does. I am quiet and have stopped shivering. I am good now. A good girl. He says I'll be fine. When he touches my forehead I notice a throbbing—I must have banged it. My mother tells the doctor I was delirious and fell from bed. Even though I can't open my eyes I nod, yes, this is true. If given truth serum I would still confirm her statement. For it is true. I was delirious, have been delirious since floating to the floor of the pool. But my temperature must have broken, he says, as I have no fever now. I'll be as good as new by morning.

My mother says I caught the flu at the pool and that if I'm not careful I will catch something worse. By now, I think I must almost believe her. Really, what is wrong with me might as well be called flu, because it has no other name for identification. It could be called flu. It could be called strep throat, leprosy, tuberculosis, leukemia. Perhaps I have them all. Surely it is something that gnaws my body. Why should the name matter?

□ □ □

It is dusk when our group arrives at Palisades Amusement Park, spinning with neon color. We eat hot dogs, cotton candy, caramel apples, while wandering around Ferris wheels and roller coasters. But it is Celeste who devours cotton candy. It is Celeste who is intoxicated by gaudy lights, by the tinny sound of music, by the whirl of rides, by the taste of sugar. She is as enchanted with Ryan as much as I miss Christopher. And I do. For while Celeste leans close and brushes Ryan's arm, I wish Christopher walked beside me. Ryan and Celeste move quickly from games of chance to speeding rides. I want her to—I don't want her to stop.

On the Ferris wheel he kisses her, a long, round kiss. His mouth tastes of sugar, and I want this—Celeste does—wants him to kiss her and kiss her, kiss all the lipstick off her mouth. And I am grateful for Celeste, who keeps us focused on this kiss, unfocused on Christopher. In the gondola they swing from the ground up, up to the night, and she feels as if she's swinging around the sky. His heart slams against her hand, and Celeste kisses him harder, deeper, craving the power of his heart. She believes she controls it, is powerful enough to control the beat of it.

Later, she sits between Ryan's legs in a scooter car as they rocket through space like a bullet. He can't kiss her now, her back is to him, but his hands are under her shirt while she presses against his chest. Now the back of her head feels the slamming of his heart. And her power, her strength, grow. On the carousel they sit beside each other in a chariot, kissing, and he asks if he can take her out Saturday night. He has an older friend with a car and they can go to the drive-in movie in Paramus. Yes, she says, she will go. In the haunted house he places her hand on his penis while his fingers slide beneath the leg of her shorts. He whispers how much he loves her. Celeste knows what this means, knows what he wants, although he would never, never ask for it, would never believe a Glen Rock girl would know how to do it, would agree to do it, ever. Celeste, Celeste, no, I try to warn her. Stop. I don't want her to do what I know she is destined for.

She doesn't stop. She unzips his pants. Her treacherous mouth lowers over him. In a moment it is over. He is too quick for her, too easy. Then she can stop.

For the rest of the evening he doesn't look at her. And she, now without purpose or reason for being, can't hear the sound of her footsteps, can't see neon lights, can't hear rock 'n' roll music blaring from loudspeakers. Her heart drains from her body. All she is left with is that taste in her treacherous, treacherous mouth.

On Saturday night I lie rigid in the back seat of the car at the drive-in movie. There are no neon lights, no whirling rides. Celeste is not with Ryan, I am, and while I know what she can do and how she does it, I am exhausted and confused with his hand under my dress, exhausted with his mouth kissing mine, exhausted by the sound of his heart slamming. I want it to stop. He's furious I won't touch his penis. Furious I won't allow it in my mouth. Furious he's spent this money to take me to the movies. When I am finally exhausted with his fury, I put his own fury in my mouth. And then, when it is over, we can stop.

□ □ □

Our family is to drive to Londonderry, Vermont, for a two-week vacation. As we pack up the car to leave, my father is in a rage. He can't arrange the suitcases the way he wants—we have brought too much—and he arranges and rearranges the trunk while screaming at us. My sister, my mother, and I stand in the garage watching him slam suitcases. Once, my mother tells him to quiet down or the neighbors will hear, but her reprimand detonates an explosion of sound. I could stop his abuse, I know it. I know how to soften it, but he doesn't even glance at me. I lean against the cool cement wall of the garage, waiting for this trip to begin. But of course it has begun. All our trips begin in rage, and all the way to Vermont I feel it.

We stay in an inn owned by an elderly couple. My sister and I share a bedroom, and the moment we arrive I crawl under white sheets and sleep in my antique bed, exhausted from the ride. I should be able to sleep all night, but late at night I awaken, startled, thinking I hear the door creak. I am afraid to open my eyes, afraid of what I might see in the doorway, afraid of what might be moving toward me, but the sheet on my bed is not edged aside. My body is still; the bed is still. Probably I heard the springs in my sister's bed as she turned over. Kiki is a light sleeper, her breath is shallow, and for a while I listen to her, soothed by her sound, soothed by the inn's scent of apples and cinnamon and lavender toilet water. Finally I sleep as a cool, dry breeze of pines flutters white lace curtains against open windows.

In the morning my parents go to town, and my sister and I are given buckets to pick vegetables in the garden. I inch along the rows, slowly snapping tomatoes off vines, afraid I'll bruise or split one by mistake. My sister, however, blazes up and down her assigned rows, finishing quickly. When she returns to the kitchen, her bucket full, I lie back in the dirt. Above me the sky seems to be floating, and I hold onto a tomato vine and float with it, watching the clouds furl. I don't want to leave here. I want to tap maple trees for syrup in winter. I want to decorate Vermont pines for Christmas. I could pick apples all fall. Tomatoes and peas in summer. I glance at the house, up to my second-story bedroom window. Really, I want to stay here because Vermont nights are so quiet.

When I finish picking tomatoes, I head across the yard toward the kitchen. My parents, returned from town, sit on lounge chairs reading the *New York Times.* My father glances at me over the rim of the paper, his gaze following me to the door. *What will you do for two weeks, Father?*, my eyes ask him—hard. When I yank open the door I look away from him and let the screen bang behind me.

My sister sits at the kitchen table drinking lemonade. A plate of oatmeal cookies is in front of her. Kiki is already at home here, is always at home in the homes of strangers. In photographs pasted into the family album she always holds hands with men and women one only faintly remembers from distant trips, or else she leans against one edge of the photograph, leans against a stranger, while I, with my mother or father, will be on the opposite side of the picture.

I refuse lemonade and cookies, too shy to eat in front of strangers. My sister wants to go with the husband out to the barn converted into an artist's studio. He says he will give my sister a small canvas and paints. Do I want to join them? I shake my head, no. Instead, the woman shows me how to place an apple on a spiked metal machine clamped to the table. Turn the handle that turns the apple, peeling the skin. I am intrigued by this, by the long coil of apple skin that curls onto the table. One after another I peel apples that she will bake into pies. After I finish, she again offers me a glass of lemonade. This time I accept a small, small glass—maybe just a little.

After lunch I sit on the antique couch in the living room. On the far wall ancient-looking books fill bookshelves. I think about reading one but am too tired to move. A cat pads toward me, its claws clicking the pine wood floor. It rubs against my ankle, then jumps on my lap, purring as I stroke its calico back. Even now, in summer, I smell ashes from the stone fireplace. From the kitchen is the scent of apples and cinnamon. I curl next to the cat on the couch, my eyes closed, lulled by cinnamon, by ashes, by the purring cat, by the silent house. On my fingers is the scent of peeled apples and tomato vines. I fall asleep smelling this, this, with the purr purr of the cat.

I awake, startled. The cat bounds from my grasp. My father is leaning over me, stroking my arm. He says we're going to the country store. Perhaps my sister and I would like to buy souvenirs? His face is close to mine, but I hear voices in the foyer. We are not alone. I quickly sit up and run outside.

At the store my sister and I are given five dollars apiece. I examine maple sugar candy in designs of trees, sailing ships, miniature people. I inhale the scent of pillows stuffed with pine needles. Tiny log cabins are incense holders, with chimneys for the smoke.

Back in the corner, in a basket, are remnants from Christmas, and I sit on the floor to examine each item. Here I find the miniature Christmas tree. I wind the base. Blue, green, red bulbs flash as the tree revolves. It is almost five dollars, but I must have it. My sister buys an incense holder, pine-scented incense, and four pieces of maple candy.

Back at the inn my sister and I close the door to our room. She places an incense cone in the log cabin and lights it. I wind the Christmas tree and place it next to the cabin. She unwraps a candy in the shape of a whaling ship, and, I am amazed, gives me half. We lie on our beds and nibble the candy.

Perhaps she's lulled by the scent of incense, by the drowsy puffs of smoke, by the revolving tree, by the too-sweet maple candy, for she rarely confides in me, this silent, secret sister. But with no warning, not even a glance at me, she asks me why I think Daddy got mad when we left on the trip. "I *hate* it when he does that," she says.

Even though the door is shut, I quickly turn toward her—toward her short thin body barely denting her bed—believing I must warn her: *Ssh, better be quiet*. Doesn't she know he might hear her, that he hears and knows everything? Yet, watching her, I wonder: Does she need the warning? For even lying still on the bed, truly she seems neither short nor thin but rather dense and powerful. We are sisters, but how can we seem so different? For my fearless sister can ignore the rules while I'm unable to open my mouth even to warn her of them. My bold-bold sister can speak aloud the word "hate" while I would never even silently dream of hating my daddy. I am the one who must be very good, very quiet.

But wait—I am able to speak. I must repeat the only words I'm taught, all that I know. "It's wasn't that bad," I whisper to my brave sister. "He doesn't mean anything by it. We really did bring too much stuff for the vacation."

My father discovers a lake with a place to rent rowboats and says he wants to teach me to row. Who wants to go along? My mother says she's tired. My sister says rowing is too slow and boring. So my father and I drive to the lake alone. We drive in silence, the windows rolled down. The wind whips my hair. And I believe, for a moment, that I will never be brought back, will never be returned to my mother, will never again see my house in New Jersey, that my father and I will never stop racing down this country highway. Without taking his eyes from the road, he reaches over and strokes my hands clasped in my lap and tells me how good it is we're finally alone together.

The man at the lake asks how long we want to rent the boat.

"A couple of hours," my father says, taking out his wallet. "If we keep it longer I'll pay when we bring it back."

"We won't be *that* long," I say. "What about dinner?"

My father waves to me to be quiet, and I glance down at the grassy shoreline.

The man helps my father slide a boat in the water. I keep my head bent, not wanting the man to see me, knowing what he must see when he sees through my clothes to my body. He knows what my father and I will do out there in the boat, in the water. He knows why my father is taking me out there. When they call to me, I stop to tie the lace on my sneaker. My father is already seated at the oars, and the man reaches for my hand to help me over the gunwale. But I stumble, knocking one of the oars from my father's hand. He yells at me to be careful.

I sit in the rear facing my father. As he pulls the oars, the boat slides through the water. The lake is smooth, our boat the only ripple except for insects skimming. The sun feels good on my bare arms, and I kick off my sneakers to let my feet dangle overboard. The lake is cold; goose bumps shiver my thighs. My father takes long, even strokes, pulling the boat far from shore. There is the creak of oarlocks, the drip of water, the scud of clouds. A dragonfly floats on a leaf and its iridescent wings shimmer in sunlight. I concentrate on it. On its transparent wings. On its rainbow colors. I think about being it. Not even the dragonfly, less, just a speck of its wing, an ephemeral flash of color.

My father is telling me a story from his childhood. His family of Russian peasants is from a small shtetl outside Kiev named Pavolich. Shortly after he was born there his father, drafted into the Czar's army but refusing to serve, fled the country for America, leaving his wife and children behind, until he earned enough money to send for them. My father was three when his mother, brother, two aunts, and he left Russia to join him in America. My father doesn't remember the exact course of the journey, but he remembers being in a big train station in Europe. He was overwhelmed by its immensity, by the crush of fleeing peasants. By mistake he let go of his mother's hand and was lost in this station. Some woman, a stranger, helped him find her again.

I think about this, think about this small scared boy lost in a train station. I try to imagine a Russian shtetl, but I can't. All I envision is vast distances, empty spaces.

They sailed from Bremen, Germany, on the *Prince Frederick Wilhelm,* arriving in New York, arriving on Ellis Island, on August 15, 1911. He still remembers, will always remember, the sight of New York harbor, the Statue of Liberty, how he, all the immigrants, cried. Because his father was not given time off from the dry-cleaning establishment where he worked (they later learned), he was not there to meet them. My father and his family were not allowed to leave Ellis Island without someone to claim them. They were told they must spend the night on the island. My father says his mother was terrified that his father wouldn't come for them. This happened to others on the island, also waiting. If husbands and fathers didn't fetch their wives and children, they were sent back to Europe.

My father and his mother, his relatives, spent the night in bunks set up like an army barracks. My father remembers the sweaty smell of hundreds of immigrants, the sound of babies screaming, the smell of fear. The next morning his father arrived to claim them, to bring them to New York City. In Russia, his father's name was Wolko Zidowetzky. Now, when his father comes to take them to their new home, his name is William Silverman.

I am sad. Again, I think of my father alone in the train station, in a strange bunk, wondering if he's been abandoned by his father. I think of the fear of a three-year-old child. I want to save him. I want to make him feel better.

I kneel in front of him, hugging him, my head against his stomach. I stroke his back to soothe him. The oars slip from his hands and the boat skims forward before slowing. He slides his fingers through my hair and kisses the top of my head and soon I am crying. "Daddy, I'm so sorry. I love you, more than anyone else in the world."

Without speaking, he loosens his belt. Without speaking, I bend my head toward him, knowing what I must do: heal the wound of that immigrant child. He grips my hair and the nape of my neck to show me the rhythm. Do it slow, his hands tell me, while you heal me. I want to heal him and believe my mouth will banish his fear forever.

But then he stops me. I look up, surprised. No longer do I see the small boy who's wounded. He *is* still wounded, yes, but the wound is larger now, more desperate, more adult, deeper. He wants me to pull down my shorts and sit on him. I don't want to do this. I want him to be the small boy again who doesn't scare me. "Daddy, people will see me." "Don't argue," he says. "Do it." I slide my shorts and white Lollipop underpants down to my ankles. I can't do this. I don't know how to do it. He puts my feet on either side of him, holds my hips, and pushes me down on it, tells me to fuck him. Go on, he tells me, *you* do it for once, you're old enough now. Move. The angle is awkward and my calves ache—I can't do it. My shorts are in the way. The zipper scrapes him and he slaps my thigh, telling me to be more careful. He unbuttons my blouse, is angry I'm wearing a bra, but he pulls it loose. "Daddy—" I know people are watching. I try to tell him— "Daddy, please button my blouse. Please." He doesn't. Still I don't move. Still my legs feel paralyzed. I can't do what he wants.

Finally he pushes me away. He tells me to straighten my clothes and sit back down, that he thought it might be nice to try something new, but now he sees I'm too stupid and selfish. He says no man will marry me if I don't let him teach me, but no man would want to marry me anyway. Maybe when I get older he'll marry me, he says. He'll have to—no one else will. He'll leave my mother and we will live far away from everyone.

I want him to zip his shorts, too, but he doesn't. I can't look at it—I know he wants me to, but I can't. Instead, I lean over the side and try to see my reflection in the water, the girl my father has proposed to, the girl he wants to marry. Briefly, yes, there I am—a glimpse of nose, eyes, mouth. But the image is shattered by oars, by the rush of water.

He nestles the boat beneath towering trees where the land plunges into dense growth. I don't want to go into that weedy darkness. I'll trip on knobby roots. Branches will snag my hair. I'm scared I'll get lost, scared I won't find my way out. But without speaking I follow him ashore, I undress, I lie on weeds and pine needles. Celeste grins up at him—Celeste, who always knows the right words to say to him. She always knows what he needs. She parts her legs and urges him to hurry.

The sun is low in the sky when I feel Celeste drain from my body. Her ivory-colored skin sinks into the marshy earth, and in her place my own skin is covered with weeds and mud. Her silky blonde hair molts to brown which is tangled with leaves. I want to swim in the lake to clean my body in ice-cold water, but I know there is not enough time.

The moment the bow touches the shore back by the boat rental office, I realize I'm not wearing my bra. That I don't have it. That I've forgotten it, have left it under the trees in the thicket. I tell my father we have to go back for it. Right now, I say, I must have it. We'll just turn the boat around, quickly. Please. We've got to find it.

He says he doesn't want me to wear it anyway, and I don't need it.

"Yes," I say, "but people will notice."

"Who?"

"Mother," I say. "Mother will see."

"No she won't," he says. "She never sees." He pulls the oars out of the water and stands up.

I suspect the man who owns the boats is angry we're late. I rush toward the car without waiting to hear what he says, not wanting to know how much additional money we owe for the rental, not wanting him to see me. I sit in the car, waiting. I spit on my palms in order to rub mud off my legs. I glance at my chest and I know, through the white material, you can see the outline of my breasts. I have not brought another bra, and we have another week of vacation. I can't walk around this way. It's simply not possible for me to live without it. I press my hands against my breasts to flatten them, but I can't stand how they feel and I hit them with my fists. I want to get rid of them, pound them into my chest. I want them to disappear . . . his words . . . disappear . . . It's his words, words I don't want to understand, that I am pounding, and I am out of the car and racing toward the lake. The water darkens, like mercury, into small quivers of light. I don't think I'll be able to reach that far shore, find it, but I must. My sneakers splash the water. My legs, my arms are lowering, sinking. In the distance I hear voices, but they are centuries away. I need to find my bra. I will swim to the other shore to find it.

Hands—my father's, that man's—grip my shoulders and legs. I am buried in water. As they raise me from the lake, water sloughs from my hair, my clothes, my skin, my mouth. Once they realize I'm safe the man asks what's wrong with me, anyway, what's going on here, and my father gets angry at him, tells him to leave us alone. My father picks me up and carries me to the car. Throws me in. He rolls up the windows and slaps me before gripping my head and banging it back against the seat. I want him to do this. *Crush it, Father. I want you to. Do it.* I want to feel brittle pieces of bone chip from my skull. But he will stop long before death, because he will need to do it, do it, do it all over again. And again. He says I am a whore who doesn't deserve how much he loves me, and if I ever humiliate him again he will whip every scrap of skin off my body. I should be grateful he hasn't already done this, he tells me. He releases my head, but still I feel it, pounding.

Yes, Father.

I don't need to say this aloud. He knows what I think. He knows every thought I have, feels every breath, understands every movement of my body.

Yes, Father. I am grateful.

Only you could love this cuntwhore body. You deserve to hurt it when it disobeys you or when someone notices I don't respect you. I will desire you always, Father. I will wait for you every night. You own my body. It will never, never be mine.

For the next week I will not wear a bra and no one will see. But surely I feel freer now, knowing my mother never knows what she knows, knowing she never sees what she sees.

□ □ □

By September, Christopher and Lynn have broken up. He and I are reunited. We break up. They are reunited. For three years he is a pendulum, Lynn and I fixed points of gravity waiting for him to swing our way. It would not occur to me to say, "I no longer wish to be with you." It would not occur to me to break up with him. I need him. I need his clean-smelling body. When he is with me, I believe a thin film of his white soap scent adheres to my skin.

"I'm sorry," he says to me. And yes, I see in his eyes he is. "I care for you—really. I get confused."

We stand on the sidewalk near the school yard. It is spring. It seems it is always spring when he knows he must leave me. Perhaps it is the lushness of nature that suddenly scares and confuses him. No longer does he see me in a shriveled winter body. Soon, in summer, my body will wear a bathing suit—that suit. Now I wear a cotton shirtwaist. My arms are bare. My legs are bare. No knee-socks. No stockings. If I quickly yank on a wool sweater and slacks I wonder if this would stop Christopher from leaving. If I could cloak this body. Or there must be a magical chant to be uttered, a simple teenage charm to be blessed—other teenage girls must know these charms and chants that prevent young teenage boys from walking away.

I glance past Christopher to forsythia bushes blooming in all the neighborhood yards. I can't watch Christopher not watching me, as he leaves me. In his shyness, in his discomfort, he will watch his feet or turn to watch a passing car.

"I don't know what I want," he adds. "I'm sorry."

If I looked at him I would see sunlight glint the palest hairs of his forearms. I would see his scared, innocent face. I know I am the one who scares him. For even after all this time, I believe I never truly became the suburban New Jersey girl he wanted. "That's okay," I finally say. "It doesn't matter."

And maybe this is the truth. For waiting at home, waiting for me, is my father, my father who would never walk away from me, my father who will never be scared.

□ □ □

In tenth grade my grades are poor. In eleventh grade they are worse. In geometry I barely listen as the teacher draws triangles and parallelograms on the board. The day he mentions the word "prove" is the day he loses me forever. I believe he lies about angles and measurements, for I know nothing can be proven. I know one item of clothing lost on a lakeshore would not prove what happened on that shore, would prove nothing. Dark circles under eyes can be caused by anything. Poor grades can be caused by anything. Starving can be caused by anything—anything could have caused me to do what I did with Steve and Ryan—or so I tell myself. Of course I don't consider proving to anyone what my father and I do together—I don't even consider proving it to myself. It's not clear to me that what we do is wrong. It is me.

Who *I* am is wrong. What we do is never considered logically; I have no exact means to measure what we do when we are alone together; I would never be able to prove to myself that what my father does to me is wrong.

So in geometry I rest my head on my palm and stare out the window. It is not even a stare, for that implies an aggressive action, as if I actively seek something. I do not. I remember the horizon I once watched in St. Thomas, that thin gray line at the farthest point of the Caribbean: a distance, a goal to sail toward and hopefully reach. Here, I see nothing as I gaze out the window. It does not occur to me to look forward, to search, to seek. "Future" is as difficult to prove as fact. So when I gaze out the window in geometry it could be snowflakes spinning past the window or a spring sun. It doesn't matter.

Nothing matters to me. It is my mother who insists a tutor be hired when she realizes I'm failing geometry. She is the one determined I pass, determined I get into college. Otherwise she would be embarrassed—how would she tell friends and neighbors about her stupid daughter? Who would marry a girl too stupid to go to college? So one night a week I must sit at the kitchen table with a tutor. Blankly I stare at the book and worksheets. I want to listen. I can't even pretend to listen. The tutor's voice seems beyond the reach of my ears. I imagine my sister, upstairs at her desk, deep in concentration. My mother walks down the hall to her bedroom. From the living room I hear my father rustle the newspaper. He is sleepy, anxious for me to finish. I glance down at one small isosceles triangle. Why must I try so hard to prove its existence?

□ □ □

I walk home from school in a blizzard. With my bookbag clutched to my chest and my head down, I'm walking blind, bundled in coat, hood, scarf, and boots. The wind whips my knees, bare between boots and coat, and my bangs are clumped with ice. Melodramatically, I imagine myself a Russian peasant crossing the steppes toward my father's shtetl. Perhaps the Czar's army pursues me. Perhaps there's to be a pogrom and all Jews will be slaughtered. This image causes me no fear. Rather, it is a source of excitement, which I crave. Perhaps this is why I do poorly in school: I'm bored. Nothing equals the danger of what I do at night with my father.

□ □ □

The spring before my sister leaves for college, our mother is once again sick. Kiki comes home from school earlier than usual to fix dinner. She cooks steaks and potatoes. Hamburgers and potatoes. She fixes salads. On weekends she bakes chocolate cakes. My mother eats nothing prepared by my sister, claiming she's too sick to eat. Yet when I return from school I notice she's rummaged about the kitchen. Saltine crackers and cans of soup disappear off the shelves.

The door to our mother's room remains shut, and when I press my ear to the door I hear her radio as she listens, hour after hour, waiting for the news. News is all she hears; news is all she wants to hear, surely more of a comfort to her than her family. Only in the evening, late every evening, she calls to me to give her alcohol sponge baths. I do, even though the sight of her body is awful.

When the doctor arrives she keeps the door closed and orders us not to disturb her. The way she's with him feels like a secret. After he finally leaves I glance in her room. Her pajamas are still unbuttoned from the examination. Her eyes are bright—no, almost glazed. She can't even see me. It is the doctor, I know, she's still seeing. It's the doctor, a stranger, this strange man, not her husband, to whom she exposes her body.

□ □ □

Once a week, when I walk home from school, I stop at the bakery. Although I know exactly what I want, I linger before the display cases, pretending to decide, pretending this purchase is thoughtfully considered rather than an imperative. What I buy embarrasses me because of the regularity of the purchase, because by now the sales clerks recognize me and know what I will order before I ask.

Birthday cakes.

White icing. Yellow icing. Pink icing. Chocolate icing. Blue icing. Cakes adorned with white, yellow, pink, chocolate, or blue flowers. Round cakes. Square cakes. Rectangular cakes. Pan cakes. Layer cakes. Chocolate, vanilla, orange, lemon, or coconut cakes. Written in script across the top are the words "Happy Birthday" with a blank space for a name. The first time I buy a cake I ask for the name "Kiki" to be filled in. After that I no longer bother.

The cake is tied into a white box and, whatever the weather, I carry it down Main Street to the railroad tracks. I take small steps on the crossties, following the track away from town toward a secluded spot in a clump of maples and pines. With the cake before me, I lean against the trunk of a tree. Leaves have begun to unfurl. A dusty spring sun filters through branches and glints off metal tracks. In an hour a train will speed past and I will be here to watch, sometimes placing a penny on the tracks. It is peaceful here, even with the train, for I can hear nothing else in its rattle and roar, not even the noise always disturbing my brain.

I untie the red and white string, then wind it around the larger ball I carry in my bookbag. I open the box. Today the cake is vanilla with coconut icing and pink roses. I have stolen a fork from home. The first bite is small and delicate—I try to concentrate on the flavor. I pluck off a rose with my fingers and place it, whole, in my mouth, feeling it cream against my tongue. Again I pick up the fork and cut off an edge. Then another. By the third or fourth bite I barely taste the cake, am only eating to be eating, am only eating to feel stuffed, filled up. In an hour the cake will be gone. When the train passes in an hour, I will feel drunk and dizzy on sugar.

□ □ □

When I first begin my period I don't think to tell my mother or sister. My father is the only one to notice.

□ □ □

After my sister leaves for college I sit on the bed in her room mourning her. Rarely have I been in this room. Rarely was *she* in this room, or in the house, but still I miss her. I lie on her gray bedspread surrounded by bright pink walls. On her dresser is a glass cage, empty now, from the time when she raised white mice for biology. Still, there is a faint odor of wood chips and mice droppings—this, rather than perfumy smells of a girl. I pick up a dust ball brushed against the bedruffle and extract a strand of her hair, holding it to the light. An autumn sun reveals auburn, blue, black streaks in it. For now, I wind the hair around my finger but plan to tuck it inside a book that I'll save forever.

I am scared for my sister. I think about her alone in Boston. I think about her alone in a dorm, far from her family. I believe she will miss us, will miss me. Kiki acts brave, but I have seen her still sucking her thumb. How will she be able to sleep in a strange bed in Boston? Even though she's always liked strangers, she might be scared being only with them, surrounded by them. Living with a strange roommate. Now, for the first time, I see a flicker of an image of myself not in this house with my mother and father. Never had it occurred to me that someday I might not live with them either. Nights. Alone. One night I might be alone in a bed in Boston. The feeling I have is not one of escape or freedom. It is fear. All I know is what I have. I believe my father is the only person who could love and care for me. It is the freedom itself that scares me. How would it be possible for me to control, be responsible for, be in charge of, my own body? I wouldn't know what to do with it.

My father climbs the stairs to my sister's room and walks to the window, barely glancing at me on the bed. He seems quiet and sad. I don't want him to be. I don't want him to miss my sister, don't understand how or why he would miss her, since, I tell myself, he hardly saw her anyway. A small pile of clothes my sister no longer wears is next to the mouse cage on her dresser. He picks up a blue Oxford shirt with a frayed collar and holds it.

"Daddy?" I say.

He says nothing. He turns from the window and sits in a chair. I want to yank my sister's shirt from his hands and rip it to shreds; I want to stop breathing. I unwind the strand of my sister's hair from my finger and let it waft to the floor. I want to say something to him—what? The base of my throat is frigid and I don't think I can speak. Still, I must. *Daddy?* I cross the room and kneel before him. *Daddy?* I want to say this to him, but I can't. Yet he must know what I'm thinking, for I believe he knows everything about me. I try to cuddle against his legs, but he doesn't respond. I try to nudge my hand against his fingers, but he doesn't loosen his grasp on the shirt—on my sister's shirt. A slow panic hardens the base of my spine and I think I might not be able to stand. *Daddy.* I grip his knee so tight it must hurt him, and his foot, no, his shoe, doesn't kick, no, but taps me, pushes me back from him—back, back, back away from him. And I do stand, then. Yes. I stand and turn and walk across the floor of her room, down the stairs to the living room, down the hall to my bedroom, and close the door. I sit on the edge of my bed watching the door, waiting for it to open when my father realizes it is *me, me, me.* I am the one he loves. But my door doesn't open.

I am outside on the stoop. I am in the street in front of our house. I walk down the street away from the house, but I don't know where I'm going or why. A sting of coolness pierces the evening. Lawns darken. A pale autumn moon rises. I feel the sap in the trees begin a slow descent for winter, draining from treetops and tips of branches down the trunks to the roots. I am walking toward town, passing houses where lights have just been turned on. I don't pause, for now I know where I'm going: to Christopher's.

I pass the large rock in the middle of the intersection at the edge of town. I cross the railroad tracks and continue down Main past the pharmacy, Mandee's dress shop, the bakery, People's Bank. Even if the bakery were open, I would not stop for a cake. I don't think I'll eat again for a long time. I'm not able to stop long enough to eat. My movements toward Christopher's seem not to belong to me. Even if I didn't want to go to his house, my feet would carry me there anyway. But now I'm not even sure if my feet will stop when I get there. Christopher lives past the high school, and it is night by the time I reach his house.

Abruptly, when I reach the top of his stoop, my feet do stop. Most of the lights in his house are on, but that is not the draw. I don't even want to go inside. I want, rather, to urge him outside, here, with me, urge him into the night. Make him understand night; make him understand what it means to be me. I want to corrupt him. Then, I believe, I can have him and will no longer need my father. When I ring the doorbell, his mother answers. She is surprised to see me and glances toward the street to see if I've been driven. She opens the screen, asks if I'm okay, invites me in, but I shake my head and ask for Christopher.

But I can't tell him why I've come or what I want—just that I'm taking a walk and I want him to walk with me. He says he can't. Says he's helping with his sisters. Says . . .

"I want you to come with me." My voice is loud and he steps outside and closes the door, not wanting his parents to hear me—I know this. I know I should leave. Should apologize for coming. I can't. I want too desperately something he can never give me: my self.

He keeps asking what's wrong. He asks if he can have his mother call my parents. Can he have his father drive me home? No, no, no. I can't be driven home. He is losing patience—I know this, too—know he will never speak to me again if I don't leave quickly. He is not prepared for this, for who I am, for what I am capable of doing. As the extreme of me nears him, he will step back. Usually my extreme is absorbed by my father, but now it rages out of control, and the more desperately I want him to be the one, now, to absorb and calm me, the harder he will run back and back and back. Christopher does not know who I am, but certainly he feels me.

He must go in, he says. He can't stand outside. His parents will get angry. He has chores and . . . I press my hands to my mouth and stop listening. While he steps inside his house, I walk backward down the path to the street. He shuts the door as quietly as possible to soften the blow. It doesn't matter. Now I see I've come to the wrong house; Ryan's house should have been my destination. Ryan would come out here with me. He, too, is easily captured by night, is incapable of refusing what it offers.

But my father . . . now I believe he's waiting. There's been a mistake. He didn't push me away with his foot. He didn't hold my sister's shirt rather than my hand. He didn't. He wants me, is looking for me, is in desperate need only of me. I run down streets I've just walked to get here, as deliberately as before, once again toward a house which I think will save me. It no longer matters which boy, which man, which house, for it is not truly toward anyone or anything that I run. Rather, it is away from me. I can't be alone with me because I don't know who I am. I'm too scared to know who I am. My father—all who I am is my father. I am he. And I know he will have turned on the porch light for me. My father will be by the front door waiting for me. Perhaps he's already opened the garage door in order to drive the streets searching for me. Or he'll be sitting on the edge of my bed, waiting.

The porch is dark. The living room is dark. The house is dark. I don't dare glance up the stairs to my sister's room, but rather rush down the hall to my bedroom and slam on the light. The bed is neatly deserted. I whirl against the door, closing it with a force that cracks the silence. I lock the door. Never have I locked it before; never have I been allowed to lock it. I turn off the light and sit on the bed, staring at the doorknob. At first I can't even see it, but soon a dull glint is visible. By the hour I watch it, wait for it to turn. It doesn't. The door to my parents' bedroom had been closed, but I don't know where my father is, if he's in there with her or upstairs with . . . I wind the base of the miniature Christmas tree and lights sweep the night red, green, white. The lights are a beacon, calling: *Daddy. You love to love me with these lights.* But the red-green-white wands of light fall flat against the wall and ceiling.

I tiptoe down the hall to the bathroom. I can't turn on the light, for there is nothing I could stand to see. I remove the bottle of aspirin from the medicine cabinet, shake some into my palm, then swallow one after another with a glass of water. I creep upstairs to the unfinished attic. Here the air is warm but untouched, undisturbed by my family. In its stillness I have trouble breathing. I am too used to breathing tornadoes of sound. Here, there is no flutter of air to help me, but I want none. Even through the gable vents I feel no sky and see no breeze. I am woozy in a voluminous black void and must lie on the floor to steady myself. I lie on my stomach. The floor smells of raw wood and it is this wood, only this smell of wood, that keeps me from roiling out through the vents in the gable. I smell the wood slowly. The smell comes slow through my nostrils and I have trouble letting it seep down to my lungs. I envision each molecule of my body settling like dust across the attic floor. I want to sleep. For as long as it would take me to reach the edge of the sky.

I think I am too groggy to breathe, but I am breathing. Hands are on my shoulders, yanking me. I can't open my eyes. Behind the lids of my eyes there is no slant of light, but I don't know if this is true on the outside of my lids as well. With every touch of his hands, my porous bones splinter. My wayward legs are without direction; he must carry me. And he does. I don't think he understands the distance I've traveled, for he is angry I have been lost. I don't know if I try to tell him why. But I must, because my ears hear a voice with tears sliding from its tongue. And he will hate this hate this hate this, what I must say.

So after he drops me on a bed he tapes this hateful mouth shut. For how can he love a mouth that wants to speak truth? My mouth must be stilled. My ears are stilled. I am. What does my mouth do to cause this? Maybe I try to tell him my fear that he loves my sister more, or my fear that my sister is alone in a dorm without me close to love her. But he won't hear what my mouth needs to utter. My father selects the only words he will hear and forbids all others. I am only allowed to tell him what my body wants him to do to it, tell him how strong is my desire. All other words I learn, I learn in secret, *are* secret, packed and stored in my own attic of my own mind. My nose is stuffed with the words that can't leak from my eyes or my mouth. I have trouble breathing. All I feel is an almost unconscious jolt as he rapes me back to life. And he will. Because with my father and me, what usually kills others, is what nourishes us with life.

And I know my father and I will be alone forever in this forever-and-ever life. I know this, as much as I know Christopher will be gone forever from my life. If only I could have told Christopher, if only I could have explained the true and only reason why I went to his house, why I needed him earlier tonight. *Christopher, I need you because I love you. I need you because you are quiet. I need you because you are shy.*

The next morning my father rips the tape from my mouth. The rawness of the skin stays with me, is there for days, is there whenever I look at my face in the mirror. My mouth hurts the most when I smile, and so I must smile whenever my father enters the room and beckons.

He loves my smile. Long after the skin around my lips has healed, I continue smiling.

□ □ □

I am a teenager. I love to listen to my transistor radio. I love to dance. I attend all the school dances and dance and dance and dance. My body feels free while I dance. I control what it does. So when I hear music I must move. I love Pat Boone, Paul Anka, the Everly Brothers, Ricky Nelson, Roy Orbison, Elvis Presley,

Bobby Darrin, Bobby Vinton, Frankie Avalon, and Fabian. Well, Celeste loves Elvis. I especially love Pat Boone. I see a photograph of Pat Boone with his four daughters and am drawn by how clean they look. Their clothes are without wrinkles. Their hair is without snarls. Their teeth shine straight and white. I want to be one of his daughters. I believe if he sees me he will adopt me, so I nag my mother until she buys tickets for his television show. After the show I wait in line with a copy of his book *'Twixt Twelve and Twenty* for him to autograph. When I reach him, I can't move. I can't raise my arm to hand him the book. I'm holding up the line. Finally he smiles and asks: "Is this for me?" I give it to him. He signs and returns it . . . except then I am back in the car, driving back across the bridge with my mother, heading toward home. Later, in my room, I trace my finger across his signature and dream about being with him, dream about being one of his daughters. And so, finally, I *am* one, asleep in his house, tucked into a clean white bed.

But when I wake the next morning I'm still in my own house. My own bed. I go to breakfast wearing red Lollipop underpants. Nothing else. My mother says nothing. My father says nothing. All day I don't dress. When my father comes home from work I'm sitting in the living room in my red Lollipop underpants. When my mother calls us to dinner I walk into the kitchen still in the underpants. No bra, no slip. Even the soles of my feet are bare. We eat our dinner like this. I don't remember whether we speak or not. Probably my father tells us about the successes of his glorious, glorious day.

* * *

But still I believe I'm a teenager like my friends. I learn to drive a car. I love the Beatles and watch them on *The Ed Sullivan Show.* I buy records. I dress like my friends. I talk like my friends. Because all I've ever wanted is to *be* a suburban New Jersey teenage girl like my friends. It is this girl, this teenage girl (yet, objectively, a *pretense* of a teenage girl, a facsimile) who finally graduates from high school, like her friends, and prepares to leave home for college.

So I am to leave home, after all. Over the summer, a summer that will be the last summer, the last time I ever live in the same house with my parents, my father knows he is losing me, losing his teenage girl. He does what he can to hold me, to make my body his forever, because he must know what will happen to me in college, must know I will have sex with other men. Maybe he knows I will truly become the girl he's made me. So he hurts me and loves me and must hate the love—and love the hurt—until I don't understand why so much had to happen to that part of my body.

By the end of summer I have bled into a red glass ornament on the miniature Christmas tree. I can't get out. My mind turns to glass, too hard, too opaque, to shatter. No one can see in it; no one can see me inside it. No one knows me or has ever known me. Even if I pressed my body against the glass and pounded my fists, I would not be able to crack this strangely protective glass. For really, I've lived inside this glass for years; the glass has only grown stronger over the years. It will protect me until I'm ready to understand what happened, ready to *feel* what happened. Until I'm ready to let someone, anyone, see me. Until I'm ready to come out. It will be years before I'm ready.

So most truly, then, I am not the one who goes to college in Boston. All anyone will know is all anyone has ever known, a pretense of a girl, who *does* look, who *can* look, like all you other girls. It is this pretense of a girl who lives in that first dorm at 199 Marlborough Street, who sleeps in that dorm bed and in all the beds that will follow, beds I sleep in alone or with others, all the beds away from the ones I shared with my first lover, my father.

□ □ □

Now, finally, I am in this first bed in which I sleep away from my father. This first night. I am in a dorm. Far away from home. In a building full of girls. A girl shares my room, and this first night I can't sleep, am too conscious of her, my roommate, conscious of all the girls on the hall and on the other floors, all these girls in one building, sleeping. There are no men in the building. I sense my roommate, this strange girl in my room, breathing, sleeping, dreaming. A stranger. Where is my father? He's not here. He's not here. He's not here. I don't feel sad. I don't feel happy. I don't feel. I don't feel *me*. I don't know who I am or what will become of me, here in this dorm of girls in Boston. I feel too light, even in this heavy brick building in Back Bay, even with the weight of all these other girls close around me. I am too light. Without my father's weight on my body, I can float through the bricks and past the girls into the night. And I do. Because for years, before I discover sanity, this escape is most truly only a return journey back home to *find* him, to replace him, until I learn how to stop.

Tonight I wonder where you are, Father. Tonight I wonder what you are doing. Do you sit alone in my bedroom waiting for me, mourning me, missing me? Do you now grasp a discarded piece of my clothing, wishing you grasped me instead, wishing I were home instead? Do you sleep in my bedroom, sleep in my bed? Tell me, Father, how do you live without me? Tonight, do you think about me, too?

BLUE

Tuesdays

H*ow can I help you?* Randy had asked.

Change me, I think. Is that the answer? Stop me. Or teach me new words, I think. Maybe that's the answer. Teach me to speak. Help me find a soul. Help me find my body. Teach me to cry.

When I first see Randy, when he first asks this question, it is the mid-1980s. Over the years I have sought help from ten therapists. Randy is the eleventh. He must be the one who will finally be able to help me.

Twenty years have passed since I first noticed the word—noticed the word "incest," yet still I can't say it, even to Randy. I saw the word almost by chance, in conjunction with the movie *Phaedra*. When I saw the word my gaze hesitated. It stopped. Couldn't flow along the line of words preceding and succeeding it. My breath stopped. My heart stopped. My throat was cold and my mouth rigid. But why—since I had never seen the word before, never read the word before, never heard the word uttered? I didn't know what the word meant, yet it stopped me like a slap.

I looked it up in the dictionary. At first I read and reread the definition, but I didn't allow myself to understand any of the words used to explain it. I didn't know what I was reading. I had to look up each word in the definition. As soon as I looked up each word

I forgot its definition and had to look it up again. I had to write each word, and the definition of each word, on a sheet of paper. "(1) Sexual. Union. Between. Persons. Who. Are. So. Closely. Related. That. Their. Marriage. Is. Illegal. Or. Forbidden. By. Custom. (2) The. Statutory. Crime. Committed. By. Such. Closely. Related. Persons. Who. Marry. Cohabit. Or. Copulate. Illegally. [Middle English, from Latin *incestus,* unchaste, impure.]"

Copulate. "To engage in coitus. [Latin *copulare,* to fasten together, link.]"

My father and I are fastened together. We are linked.

I feel a revulsion I don't understand when I see the word "copulate." The three short, hard syllables slam against my teeth as I whisper the word over and over. I feel a fear I think I understand too well when I see the words "illegal," "crime," "forbidden." A crime has been committed. I know I'm responsible. I've committed unpardonable sins. But I don't understand what the sins are. I have these words written on a piece of paper. I will be punished for these words. But I don't know why.

I see the movie. I watch a mother and a son in bed together. That night, all night, I feel my father in bed with me. Yet he is not with me. My body only feels as if he is. I feel as if he's exploding through my body, my throat, and into the roof of my mouth. Then I am in the bed with Phaedra and her son. They hold me down while my mother slices off my nipples and staples every part of me shut. My father comes to me, stabs them, sews my nipples back on, and rips out the staples. My mother is dead. And he, my father, and I live "in a sexual union between persons who are so closely related that their marriage is illegal or forbidden . . ."

"We are forbidden," I whisper to my father. And he laughs.

Days later I can pretend the word and the movie don't exist. Or dictionaries and movies lie. With equal ability I can also pretend the word and the movie have nothing to do with me, nothing to do with what happened to me with my father. This movie, this word—more—my childhood—my memories—sometimes, yes, they are like snapshots, glimpsed images. Memories are also like the ocean, like tides in the sea. Memories roll close to me, curled in the scroll of a wave, suddenly revealed when the wave crashes ashore. Then the memory ebbs, flowing out to sea. Memories tugged back and forth by the moon, memories of what happened at night with my father.

But never does the ocean evaporate. So never can I forget. What I most lack is understanding. I don't understand what happened to me because I don't understand the darkness of the deep, mysterious sea.

I don't understand this darkness, this mystery, because I know no words to decipher it. To ensure I never do, there are moments of time when I don't allow myself to see words, when I can't see *any* word, for any word might reveal a truth I don't want to know. So for days after seeing the movie, I'm unable to read even one word with ease. None. I can't read magazines. I can't look at billboards or street signs. If I fill the car with gas I can't read the name of the station or how much the gas costs. When I write out a check I am filled with anxiety at the words on the printed check. I can't glance at the mail. I can't look up a number in the phone book, but, then, there is no one to call. I can't read the words on a package of food. As long as I am wordless I will not know the truth of the sin I have committed.

□ □ □

Randy, how can you help me? Before I can whisper that word "incest," I must whisper the name of a man who just exploded through my life and left me speechless, a man who, although he's not a child molester, reminds me of my father. Over the years since I left home there've been too many men, so many names I could whisper to Randy.

But Tom is the name of the man now.

The moment I see Tom I understand him. He is married. *I* am married—to Mack, a sweet, shy man who scares me, scares me because he might actually love *me*, not just my body. With Tom, who can destroy me, I feel no fear, for he is familiar. He is the archetype of the dangerous man, the original myth of the man who destroys women's hearts and bodies. He is the fury and rage of every man I have fucked, the mentor of every man who causes danger and grief. Only my father commands more rage. *But, Tom, don't you know? This is why I select you: Because you are no longer human—because you have lost your own soul, surely you are the only one capable of loving the soulless body my father created.*

But he doesn't love me. In a fury of lies he betrays me. Now, now—knowledge is only a glimmer—I begin to see, I begin to know, that mute sex isn't love. It has never, ever been love. The rage I feel shatters the protective glass walls in which I live. It shatters me. Without this glass scaffold, rage implodes and I am immobilized, terrified, exhausted.

June. July. My husband is away for the summer, and I am alone. Week after week, after being with Tom, I want to be alone—I must be. For I don't want anyone to see. Me. When the last chip of glass falls to my feet, I don't want anyone to see this soulless girl, stripped and exposed. If my husband knows who I am—if anyone sees who I really am . . .

It is August, and hot. I lie in bed in the upstairs bedroom. Sweat drips down my body. I can't take a shower. I can't clean myself.

For fifteen years I've had a cat, and this cat is now dying of feline leukemia. My cat is too sick to climb the stairs, even though he needs comfort. Below me, through the floor, I feel my cat dying and I can't save him. I can't give him comfort, even though I've loved him longer than I've been able to love any human. Once a day, at dusk, I edge down the stairs and manage to put a few chips in his bowl and give him a little water. He is too sick to eat, and for a long moment I sit on the kitchen floor beside him. I want to save him, I want to cure him, I want to comfort him. I can't. I stroke his chin and hear the thinnest of purrs—at least, yes, he's still purring. I don't want him to stop. It is this purr. And her. The girl I left behind on the beach in the West Indies. Her. I can't see her, that girl, but there is something. A piece of a fingernail. One strand of hair. One heartbeat of hers that keeps beating. But then the kitchen, the linoleum floor, the downstairs of the house, scare me, and I must go back upstairs to bed.

The first month after I have sex with Tom my period is unmanageable. I dream a penis is a knife disconnected from a body, stabbing me. When I wake, the sheet is bloody. At first I don't recognize the blood as menstrual. No, it's the evil that lives inside me. What I did with Tom is evil. Sex is evil. And Tom is sex. I feel the blood beneath my torso, staining my skin like a tattoo. I run my palm across it and know I am drowning in blood. I feel it bubble from my mouth and nostrils. With Tom, his danger is as dark as the stain on the sheet, and my body feels this danger for the first time. Or, I *allow* myself to feel danger for the first time . . . because long ago I abandoned all feelings and never allow myself to feel anything.

But wait, no, I am wrong: It's *not* the first time I feel danger. Truly, the sight of blood on sheets—this feeling of terror it causes—is familiar, because this is really the second time I have felt it. It's only now that I *recognize* it, begin to understand for the first time that terror and danger are not synonyms for love. Terror is not the definition of love. Tom's sexual rage is the conduit to the past, the nightmare to reawaken me to my long incestuous sleep. Because of Tom I'm able to *decipher* the nightmare, a nightmare that could never be named "love." Because Tom is terror, I remember him as well as my father. I remember both of them.

But I don't want to remember terror. I want to forget. One evening I think I must eat and eat and eat in order to help me forget it. I must eat until I'm too stuffed to think, too dense to remember. I rush from my bed, my body moving faster than I am able to, and I almost trip going down the stairs to the kitchen. I have trouble grasping pans, flour, cinnamon, sugar, the round carton of oatmeal—my hands moving quickly, my heart slamming—yet knowing, yes, I must eat oatmeal cookies. My eyes move too quickly to read ingredients, and I'm tossing stuff in the bowl that may or may not belong, in proportions that may or may not be accurate. It doesn't matter. I must eat and eat, gorge myself on oatmeal cookies. I mix the ingredients with my hands and drop gobs of batter onto a greased cookie sheet. I slam the pan into the oven and wait. I can't wait. I don't want to wait. I feel as if I'm caught in a tornado that can't stop, and I want to eat the cookies now. I have brought my supply of razors with me and to comfort me while I wait I sit on the floor and cut my legs, my thighs, cut myself in that nameless part of my body until I bleed onto the tan linoleum floor. My cat pads over to me while I wait for the cookies to bake.

I place the pan of cookies on the floor. In order to forget I must eat them all, so before they are even cool I stuff them in my mouth. I must fill myself now. There is no time to chew. I swallow clumps of dough barely cooked. It had not occurred to me to time them. There was not enough time to time them. I put a few small pieces in front of my cat. Maybe the cookies will help him, too, but he doesn't eat them. And when I've finished all the cookies in the pan, I pick up those crumbs and eat them, too.

When I finish I lie back on the floor. My heart begins to slow. I'm moving slower now. I press my hand to the linoleum. It is still. The oatmeal cookies, heavy in my stomach, root me to the floor. My cat curls up beside me, his head against my arm, and I want to stroke him. But then, then, I'm unable to lift my hand or even move it. He purrs anyway, and I'm lulled by the sound. I don't want him to stop. I want to drift away on his purr, purring. And I do.

The phone startles me awake—my father calling . . . his voice tracking the scent of blood here to the kitchen floor. How can he speak words to ears that aren't human? How can he penetrate a mind that's now numb? How can I respond to him with a mute mouth, that mouth he taped shut? He plans to write a book, he is saying, this man who's now retired and is anxious by time he now believes to be empty. Except, he tells me, in a voice he believes I could never refuse, he really thinks *I* should be the one to write the book, a book about his career with the Trust Territories. "Of course we'll work on it together," he says. "Our special project."

"I don't know anything about the Trust Territories," I barely whisper.

"I've been telling you about them for years."

I never listened.

"Just come up here. I have notes. I need you to do this." Besides, he says, he and my mother have a free trip to Venice, but my mother's too sick to go. Will I care for her while he goes? This would be a good opportunity to begin the book.

"No," I whisper.

No.

This is all I can whisper, just this one thin syllable. No. Finally, no. *I can't do what you ask, Father. No. I can't. I can't care for my mother, I can't write your book, Father. No.* Yet I am weeping, and the more I cry the angrier he becomes because I'm unable to comfort him, because I refuse to write his book. He yells at me to stop crying. "I want you to be like always," he screams at me. "Can't we just be the way we've always been?"

No, Father, I can't. No.

My mother gets on the phone, her voice feeble, asking me to come, just a few days. By now I can no longer say the word "no." Surely her feverish senses would prevent her from hearing me anyway. Surely she's too sick to notice me here on the linoleum floor, thin as a Gillette single-edged razor. Surely she's too ill, has always been too ill, to protect me from his anger, shield me from his rage. Surely the disease she suffers is loyalty to her husband. *So, Mother,* I want to say to her, *if you're so loyal to your husband, why don't you write his book?*

Then I must I must I must slam down the phone.

But, Daddy, don't you know? I *am* the way I've always been, believing dangerous men like you truly love me, that they show me how much they love me with sex. I pause on the threshold of my father's house, never truly leaving him, never leaving home, in a perverse way remaining faithful to him, faithful to the lessons he taught me. Faithfully, I repeated all the lessons, duplicated all the patterns I learned growing up, always seeking a shy man like

Christopher, like my husband—while Celeste always craved a predator lover like Tom. *And like you, Father.*

At the last minute, when she realizes I'm not coming home, my mother's illness disappears and she goes to Venice.

No one writes my father's book.

□ □ □

It is autumn. My husband, a college professor, returns from California where he's been doing research. He is tall, tan, healthy. I'm awed by the expansiveness of his health, while he is awed by my containment of such illness and filth. He must be horrified by this woman. Who is this woman he has married?

My cat has lost almost all muscle tone. No longer can he jump on his favorite chair to watch birds, so I pick him up and place him by the window. For hours I sit beside him and stroke him. I feed him milk and shrimp dinners. He eats little. His fur that once smelled warm now smells sickly. My cat has been with me longer than any man, and I don't want to lose him.

But the vet says it's time to say good-bye. He asks if I want to stay with my cat while he injects him. Yes, yes. I must be with him. I hold his paw and stroke him, telling him I love him. I tell him how bad I feel that I offered him no comfort over the summer. Perhaps he understands. He lies so still, his eyes staring—what does he see? Does he know? I want him back. I want to be able to tell him again and again what he's meant to me. I sit on the floor in the corner, weeping. I believe I will never stop missing my cat.

The vet puts my cat in a box and I bring him home. My husband digs a hole in the garden, and we bury him with his bowls and his blanket. I sit beside the grave for hours, the October dusk cool on my face. In November I plant tulip bulbs around his grave. In the spring they bloom, red and yellow. I know my cat sees them. I believe my cat loved me, too.

I hope I was a good mother to my cat, too. Except I fear I was overprotective, never allowing him outside. So why do I never have children? Surely the same reason. I see children on the street, or my sister's children, friends' children, and what I first envision is not the joy of children but rather all that can harm them. Mayhem. Devastation. I would never be able to let a child—*my* child—out of my sight either. Someone might harm her. I am overwhelmed by fear, by all that can happen to a small child. Even though I never associate these fears with what happened with my father, maybe I never have a child because I would always fear her grandfather.

□ □ □

To Randy, I bring small offerings of who I am. Tuesday after Tuesday, month after month, I reveal to him the shambles of my childhood, the shambles of my life. Entering his office I enter a holy temple of pure, rarefied air, and I feel as if I have been blessed to be allowed to breathe it.

Yet at first the offerings I bring are small, poor. Because with as much vehemence as I believe his office is a safe place, the place I should be, the place I must return to week after week in order to heal, with equal vehemence I doubt what I know to be true: I don't trust this man who is the most trustworthy man I have ever known.

So with as much determination as I arrive at his office, over an hour from my home, with equal determination I want to flee, want never to come back. But every week I am back.

When I first enter his office, I close the shades to block the light. I don't want him to see me. I'm afraid I'll scare him. I'm afraid to let him know who I really am. For if I truly let him know *me,* I believe he will leave me. I'm also afraid my body smells and that it shouldn't even be allowed to sit in his office, contaminate the rarefied air. Once he realizes how disgusting I am, how disgusting my body is, I believe he won't allow me back. Still, every Tuesday I bring to him another tiny memento of my life, and every Tuesday he makes another appointment for me to come back.

Sometimes, during a session, I'm afraid to speak because truth can sound too scary. Instead, I write him a note on a small scrap of paper: *I don't know how to tell you what's wrong.*

He writes back: *You'll talk when you're ready. No one ever taught you to speak, when everything in the world was wrong.*

I take the pencil and the scrap of paper: *Help me.*

I'll always be here, he writes. *Let me help you.*

I study the scrap of paper. *I'll always be here.* He will always be here. His patience is infinite as he waits for the snapshots—those snapshots—to surface from my secret mind. Quietly he looks at them, every Tuesday, takes them from me one at a time, replacing them with new snapshots—no, with long-lasting photographs of a woman healing. And every Tuesday I try to paste these new photographs in my mind and believe this healing woman is me.

"I'm ashamed," I finally whisper, revealing these two words as if they're gifts of string, a piece of biscuit, a stub of candle, or a wilted flower carried over a vast arid distance before finally being placed at a shrine. At the shrine even poor offerings are blessed, the bearer healed.

"It's not your shame," Randy says. "It's your father's. Give it back to him, where it belongs."

"But it's *my* body. My body is disgusting."

"No," he says. "What your father *did to you* was disgusting. You're not. Your father raped you."

"But I must have seduced him. That's all I know how to do."

"Incest isn't about sex," he says. "It's about power and control. You had none. All you were was a child."

"But what about now? Who am I now?" I feel as if my body is tattooed in men's fingerprints. These skin-deep marks are all that I am. Nothing has penetrated the surface. I feel empty. I don't think anyone lives inside me. "I don't believe I'm human," I whisper.

"You are," he says. "You're very human."

I look at this man to determine whether he might be lying. Even in his darkened office his face is the color of a copper penny. The hair on his arms glistens. I see him full of sun, full of light.

"Your father raped you." At first I struggle to understand Randy's words. What does he mean when he says the word "rape"? What does he mean when he says the words "pedophile" and "child molester"? He says these words but I can't understand them. *Let me help you,* he'd written on that scrap of paper. Yes, this is why I'm here. I must let Randy teach me.

But I must do much more than merely show him those snapshots, just as he does much more than merely see them. Randy helps me because he teaches me the words that decipher what those snapshots, those images, mean. I must now learn true definitions for words such as "rape" because I've known no words, no symbols, no definitions, to explicate the images of what happened with my father. Growing up, I didn't want to know those words, because if words for acts didn't exist, the acts themselves didn't exist. So I had no context in which to view the images: I never understood what I saw; I didn't want to understand what I saw.

Now, I must learn to substitute one reality for another, one vocabulary for another. For "seduction," Randy teaches me I must hear the word "rape." For "My father really loved me," I must hear "Your father was a pedophile and a child molester." I stop breathing when he says these words, so maybe I do understand them. Or *she* does. Randy says there's a small, wounded child who lives inside me. Months pass before I realize he is talking about the girl on the beach, the girl I thought I left behind.

"She's the keeper of your feelings," he tells me. "All those unfelt feelings are still inside you. To heal, you must feel them now. The pain of what happened."

Pain.

To me, the word "pain" means razor blades and rape, pain that my father taught me was pleasure. I don't tell Randy. I would feel shame if he knew what I'm thinking, for this can't be his definition. Randy means emotional pain, of course. But these words are hollow. The words "emotion" and "feelings" are hollow. I could look them up in the dictionary, but still I wouldn't know what they mean. I can't attach them to a tangible entity that has anything to do with me.

I look at Randy but say nothing. The intensity of his blue-blue eyes is softened by the tender skin beneath them. It crinkles when he smiles, but I don't want him to smile at me. I don't want him to like me. I don't want to like him. I'm terrified I'll love him—because love means only one thing to me. I don't want to have any feelings toward him at all. So I'm scared to think of him as a man, or even human. I feel safest when I think of him as a sprite or a spirit, awaiting the long line of grown-battered children. We silently slip inside his door, palms out, handing him our own small bits of string and wilted flowers from our tattered lives, these offerings, to be blessed or exorcised. Randy will help us.

□ □ □

I have an eating disorder and a sexual addiction. With food, I'm mostly anorectic, addicted to starvation in order not to feel, to numb-out. I watch my body grow thinner than light. No one can touch it or see it. It's a gray wisp, barely visible, refracting particles of light. I have no limbs, no torso, no heart, no stomach, no mouth. I can sleep inside a leaf or between petals of a flower. My body becomes a curl of wind. Yet if I *am* the wind, I command the leaves and flowers, direct their course. By starving, I believe I am strong, not weak. I am the only one who can control what I will eat. I am the only one who will control the fate of my body.

"You sexualize food," Randy tells me. "It's not uncommon with incest survivors."

Incest survivors. Those words don't apply to me. I don't mind having an eating disorder or a sexual addiction—that sounds all right. In fact, I'm grateful for the label. The label allows me a definition—this is who I am. I have a disease I can work to control, not so different from being an alcoholic. My drug of choice is food; my drug of choice is sex. But I hate the word "incest." The word sounds like "nest of snakes." And I don't know what it is I've survived. Incest/Celeste. I wonder if she and Dina will survive.

"If you stop eating, if you don't have a body, you can't have sex," Randy says.

"I love sex," I say, lying. I glance at him to see if he believes me. He's watching me, never fails to watch me, his eyes always forgiving, even when I say something that could never be true.

"Most sex addicts I work with hate it," he says. "The addiction has nothing even to do with sex. It has to do with fear of getting close. Or intimate."

Yes, I'm terrified of intimacy. To keep men from truly seeing me, from truly knowing me, all I speak are words of seduction, words my father taught me, words of emotional isolation. These words keep men at a distance, as far away from who I really am as possible. I never learned how to be intimate with anyone; I never learned how to be intimate with myself.

"How do you feel after?" he asks.

After. I know he means after sex. After I was with Tom I felt bereft. I think of the word "inanition," but I'm not sure exactly what it means. Later, when I get home, I look it up in the dictionary: "Exhaustion, as from lack of nourishment. The condition or quality of being empty." After I was with Tom I felt soulless, spiritually empty.

"Sex for a sex addict is a temporary high," Randy says, "like getting drunk."

Yes, in the addiction I spiral in inverted gyres, from the temporary, escalated high of sex to the downward spiral after. To inanition. The plunge is steep. For after I have sex I feel hungover. "After—" I say, "after, I feel as if someone has died." And so need to feel high again quickly. Again and again.

"*She's* the one who feels as if she's died," he says. This little girl who lives inside me, who Randy calls my "inner child." "*That* kind of sex—with that kind of man—will kill her."

I nod. I know this is true. I'm addicted to these men, addicted to danger, addicted to destruction, addicted to the death these men offer. What I've never been addicted to is life.

"Every time you have sex with one of those men, you're having sex with your father. Let him go," Randy says.

I'm scared. I know who I am with these men; I don't know who I am without them. I believe I am nothing without them.

"You're okay now," Randy says. "You'll *be* okay. You're safe. Your father can't hurt you anymore. You're strong enough to say 'no.'"

I watch him, wondering who he sees when he sees me.

"You know how to stop," Randy adds. "Let yourself feel the pain. Stop running from it. Feelings can't kill you. It's these men. They're the ones who'll kill you."

"I want them to," I say. I believe I mean this.

"But you must save *her,*" he says. "You must."

Her. That girl.

"She needs you to heal her. She needs for you to care for her, even if you can't care for yourself."

I nod at him. I feel tears, but they're not my tears—not mine—*hers?* The girl's. Yes, I begin to see her, although she's not yet distinct. At first all I clearly see is her arm and one thin shoulder. As I look more closely, I notice a small bruise on the shoulder. I realize I am the one who must care for this arm and this shoulder. But I'm not ready. She scares me. I'm afraid once she starts crying she won't be able to stop.

I glance away from Randy, toward the black and white Ansel Adams photograph on the far wall. It is of water, of a lake, of mountains. In the motionless, always present tense of the photo, nature is still. In this stillness I believe I inhale pure air of vast distances. I am a silent crust of snow, never melting; I am the surface of water on the lake, forever unrippled; I am a boulder on the mountain, still as stone, removed from a scary world of movement and feeling and noise beyond the photograph's boundary, beyond its frame. I am isolated. Cool. Alone. I want to believe I am only safe when I am alone. I glance back at Randy. But I can't be alone.

His eyes tell me this as if he can read my thoughts, even as he says nothing. I can't be alone. Not if I want to get better.

Yet still I believe I don't know how to get better. For with no warning I can crash outside the frame of that photograph, destroy the peace of that scene, the peace of Randy's office, the peace of my home. With no warning or comprehension, I rage at Randy, or at my husband, determined to frighten each of these gentle men far away. I do this until my husband tells me he barely knows who he is anymore: he feels he's losing himself, because I am like an out-of-control storm destroying everything.

Before I destroy him, I must make my husband leave me. I yell at him to rape me. I yell at him to kill me—in my craziness believing these are the words I must say in order to scare him away. I hear myself say these awful words believing the words will save him, save me, and I don't know how to stop myself from saying them.

One morning when I am screaming at him and crazy he slams his fist into a mirror. I wish he had slammed his fist into me, but this man, my husband, would never do that. I tell him he has to leave me—now—or I will end up killing us both. I fill a bathtub with water and sit in it, pounding my fists and crying. With a Gillette single-edged razor, I cut the only place on my body that doesn't exist, that I can neither name nor know. I don't think I have a choice. I must bleed. I am mesmerized by blood, as addicted to blood as is my father. I cut myself because I believe I'm evil. I have always believed I must punish myself by bleeding. I believe my blood is this evil and he, *he* is the one who owns the blood. I must drain it from my body. I never feel pain as I cut my body. My body is nothing. I don't even live inside it. Why must I lug it around, this burden of a body, always too heavy, even when it's skinny? I know this body deserves to die. Soon it will be leached a pure transparent white. It is only then I'll be able to love it.

Finally, I am calm—calmer. Thin swirls of blood waft through the water. It is my belief that blood calms, that after I cut myself, after I drain evil from my body, I am better. Simply, I exhaust myself and am depleted. Now the house is silent. My husband has gone to the hospital for his injured hand, and I force myself to breathe deeply, to concentrate, be calm. I focus on an image I know will calm me. My usual fantasy, my usual image: isolation. Escape. To get in an old rusty car and drive till it breaks down, drive anywhere. I will live in a room in a rooming house with a plastic lace doily from Woolworth's on the coffee table. I will sleep in a bed where only strangers have slept. I think of a greasy indentation on a graying pillow and know this is where my own head must be. I want to lean my elbows on a windowsill and feel all the strangers' elbows that have leaned there before. This is all I want to feel. This is the closest to anyone I want, ever, to be. To be totally alone, cool and distant, is the only way to be.

But Randy . . . in my head I hear Randy whispering. Finally someone remembers my true name and calls to me: *Sue, come home. It's time to live with safe people. There are people who care for you now.*

Randy cares for me now. And I know, I know, I care for him also. His blue eyes. His copper-colored skin. He usually wears blue. The two couches in his office, as well as the walls, are also blue. So it is these colors—copper and blue—that must mean warmth and safety. It is these colors, rather than the frost of isolation, I must remember.

Randy is frightened when I tell him I cut myself. This surprises me, because I feel no fear at all. When he says I must go into the hospital if I even think about cutting myself again, I tell him I had to do it because I'm evil.

"What your parents did to you was evil," he says. "That doesn't make *you* evil."

"My blood is," I say.

"No," he says, "your blood isn't evil. Your fear of it is your shame. It's a symbol. To you, the blood is how you both feel and see your shame."

Shame. The long syllable of the word slowly sluices through my veins. The word stains me, irrevocably. He is right. The strength of my shame stains me with the irreducibility of blood. Yet the moment he says it I feel it, and then, for that moment, it is no longer blood. It is sad. I am sad.

"You cut yourself so you don't feel your feelings," he says.

"They feel too big."

He nods. He understands. He understands everything I tell him.

"If you take care of me I won't have to do this stuff again," I say.

He tells me I must learn to take care of myself. That I must be an adult and accept responsibility for myself and for her, the little girl—that she needs an adult to care for her.

I tell Randy I'm ashamed I'm an adult who acts like a child, that I can't seem to learn skills other adults possess. "I just want . . . I want you to teach me."

"I am."

But this isn't what I mean. I want him to accept full responsibility for me. I want to be a child again. I want him to raise me, adopt me, hold a little girl hand and take me to the zoo. "Maybe if I could just live on your front stoop," I say. I am serious. I don't smile saying this.

I see this, yes. If I could live on his front stoop, close to him, then maybe I would be safe.

He smiles at me—but kindly. I won't smile back. That my anger is unreasonable doesn't matter to me, because my desire for him to adopt me is too great.

□ □ □

By chance I say the word "pedophile" in Randy's office. I have never called my father this before. I accept that the word and the condition exist, but not within my father. After the three awkward syllables have been spoken, I forget the rest of the sentence to which the word is attached. I say nothing. I wait. I wait for something to hurt my body. For something will hurt it, I'm positive.

Randy is in his usual position, leaning back on his couch, his notebook on his lap. "How does it feel to say that word?" he asks.

How does it feel, how does it feel? "I don't know how it feels," I say. "Why does everything have to feel?"

"You sound angry," he says.

"Fine, then," I say. "Angry."

Always, he asks how I feel. How does everything feel? His goal is for me to attach feelings to events, to words, to thoughts, to conversations. Everything must have a feeling. Randy has a list: *Mad, sad, glad, scared.* As on a multiple-choice test, I must select a word from his list and connect it to a feeling that is connected to me, now connected to a specific word I have uttered. I'm sick of feelings. I'm sick of trying to figure them out. I want to sing the song "Feelings" to him, somehow wonderful in its thinness, its absolute lack of feeling. But I won't let myself joke with him. For me, joking, kidding is more intimate even than telling him how I feel.

Am I angry at the word I have spoken? No, no, no, I am scared. Driving home from his office I develop a sore throat. By the time I reach home I have laryngitis. The word hadn't left my mouth, after all. Rather, it lodged in my throat. By the next day I no longer remember the word at all. All I remember is that there's a word beginning with the letter *P* that scares me. I can't remember the letters that follow.

□ □ □

A raging summer storm uproots scores of trees near my house. For days, work crews cut branches and trunks in order to cart off debris. Chain saws rip bark until I believe I feel the wet, heavy pulp on my skin. Sap sticks to my thighs. If I follow the scent of this pulp I will follow its trail back to my father. To our first house in Washington. To the sound of his saw. To the smell of sawdust and cut wood. I once felt the blade of the saw drawing closer and closer to wood. I felt the first nick in the wood, the pierce of steel, the unrelenting slice, the sap oozing from the wound, while my shoulders remained clamped in the vise. I think I feel this now, the blade cutting my body, and I call Randy. No, no, he tells me, it was then. This can't happen now. It was back then.

But it doesn't feel as if it's back then. By next Tuesday, when I see Randy, I imagine the little girl is emaciated and naked. I imagine I carry her in my arms while her head lolls listlessly against my shoulder. I tell him she is dying. I can't save her. She is too sick to be healed. Her skin is bruised and bleeding, the surface of her eyes already dead.

I curl up on the couch in his office and place her on the floor by his feet. "You take care of her," I tell him. "I can't."

He tells me to close my eyes and he will help me imagine her back to health. He tells me she must be bathed, fed, clothed. I don't want to do this. How much easier to abandon the responsibility to him. In fact, I tell him, she doesn't even exist. After all, I say, I can't see her.

"You can feel her," he tells me.

And with a slight jarring of my heart, I know this is true. It's just—I'm afraid to feel her. I'm afraid to feel what she knows. I'm afraid to feel what happened to her years ago.

Still, I close my eyes. I try to imagine. A bathroom. It is clean and white. I sit with her while I run bathwater. But she is scared to take a bath, I tell Randy. He says this time will be different. So I pour honeysuckle bubblebath in warm water. I believe she will like this scent, and we sit on the edge of the porcelain tub and watch the water foam white. I scoop up a dab of bubbles and dot her nose and her chin. It tickles, she whispers. I blow it away. We watch the slow foam curl through the air before alighting on the mound of bubbles. I smile at her. She smiles back and I think I am crying.

When the tub is full she slides beneath the bubbles. Yes, she feels safer this way, her body hidden. The room is silent. We are alone—she and I alone together—for we hear no footsteps outside the door, no hand gripping the knob, no whisper of air through the window. She holds up her arms and I wash them, smoothing a bar of soap from shoulders to wrists. She raises her legs until just her kneecaps poke above water. I rub the soap around them until they glisten. I say she has the cleanest kneecaps ever. She giggles, and the sound pops like tiny bubbles. When I try to give her the soap in order for her to wash the rest of herself, Randy stops me.

I open my eyes. What's wrong?

"She's just a little girl," he says. "You have to teach her."

"I'm not going to touch her—there," I say. "That's disgusting. She would hate it. I'll tell her how to do it. She can do it for herself."

"It was only disgusting the way your parents did it," he says. "Safe parents teach their children how to wash themselves. It's okay for you to do it. You won't hurt her."

"This is crazy," I say. "She's not even real. We're acting as if she actually exists. No one can touch her. She's just in my mind."

"I'm not going to play this out with you," he says. His voice is firm. I know he won't—nor do I want him to—although I test him endlessly. "I don't blame you for being angry," he says. "But get angry at *him*. He's the one who touched you in the bathtub."

Yes, I know. I know I must learn to get angry at *him*. How much safer, though, to get angry at Randy, because I know he will never hurt me or leave me.

But I've lost the little girl for today. I can no longer imagine her, and I'm scared I've lost her forever.

"She's not really gone," Randy assures me. "Just tell her you'll never do anything to hurt her."

Driving home from Randy's office I think of her, of children, of my sister's children. My first January in Boston I'm at the hospital when my nephew is born, and I see him moments after his arrival. A nurse brings him into a waiting room where I sit with his father. But when I see Todd, my nephew, the waiting room fades. The nurse fades. The baby's father fades. Todd is all I see. I am in awe of the small treasure of this baby. Gently, I want to touch his fingers and toes. I want to cradle his head, smooth his wispy hair, watch over him. An unfamiliar feeling, one I don't recognize, one I've never felt before, engulfs me. It is warm, it is deep, it is true. I don't have a word for it. Yet it is so strong I feel it overpowering all else that I am. It is protective, savage and primitive, ancient in its strength, as if I have suddenly grown claws of a bear and fangs of a cat. It is so primal I believe I would be able to shred any person, stop any harm, that might ever befall this baby.

□ □ □

My parents visit me and my husband. One evening, one moment really, my father sits on the bed in the guest room removing his shoes. I lean against the doorjamb, barely in the room, while we talk. During a pause in the conversation he pats the bed next to him, his gesture asking me to come to him, to sit beside him. For a moment I can't move. Nor can I say the word "no," would never be able to utter it. Finally I create an excuse—I must do something. I turn and walk away.

The next morning, again when we are alone, he comes up to me in the kitchen and puts his arms around me. He tries to kiss me on my mouth. At the last moment I turn my head, barely, almost imperceptibly, but enough so he kisses my cheek instead.

Randy is ecstatic when I tell him, Randy, who discovers success in the most minute achievement.

□ □ □

But after their visit, perhaps scared by their visit, or scared to have refused my father, I have what Randy calls body memories. Without warning, my legs feel paralyzed. I wake up in the middle of the night and feel that my hair is being pulled, pulling my head back and back until I can barely swallow. My head feels as if it's severed from my throat.

I don't want body memories. I don't want a body. So for weeks I eat nothing but cream cheese and potato chips. I believe I will be healthy with an emaciated body. I will be strong and powerful chalk white, drained of blood. For hours I lovingly caress a Gillette single-edged razor with a fingertip, feeling the seduction of cool sharp metal. I refuse to throw away the razors. I refuse to eat. Randy says I must go into the hospital for treatment.

The first three days in the unit, all I feel is rage. The therapists say I'm in withdrawal. Here, forced to eat three meals a day, I'm withdrawing from starvation. With no blood flowing out of my body, I'm also withdrawing from death. I don't want to live; my addiction doesn't want me to. This unit will attempt to get rid of my addiction, while my addiction wants to rage back in control, getting rid of me instead. In the hospital its power weakens, even though it feels like a coiled monster slumbering, waiting to strike. I must spend this month learning to dissipate its power.

One morning in the shower, the only place to be alone in the unit, I stand in the tiled stall, not wanting to leave, even though I usually hate water. I wish to live in a small, silent room like this with no windows. Outside it is summer; inside this shower it could be any season, any place, any time. Here in this shower no one can hear me or see me. In this isolation, as the water drenches me, I begin to cry.

But it's not me crying. The deep, deep sound is different. Never have I heard this before, and I know it is her crying. I am awed by the sound. I don't want these tears to stop. I know this is the first time she's cried, and all she needs is for me to be gentle. And I tell her, yes, I will try.

□ □ □

It's here in the hospital I finally learn how I inherited what my father did to me, understand *why* my father did it. It's now I learn the legacy, as Randy calls it. I have long, slightly out-of-control conversations with my parents on the telephone. I have an eating disorder, I tell them. This isn't too difficult to say. The other is: I tell them I have a sexual addiction, too. I do not mention the word "incest." I do not say to my father, *You, Father, molested me.* I say only that I was taught sex is love and that I have confused everything in my life. I do not say who taught me. I do not say where I learned this.

But does my father understand? Does he know what I'm really saying? He must. For my father—my father tells me a secret. Oh, his voice is small and frightened. Now *he* is a young boy—he is the one scared. Not so much scared to tell me, I suspect, but scared because he still believes *he* will be punished by his mother. He will be punished for telling the secret, punished because he believes it's his fault it happened. In a small, young voice he tells me his childhood secret: that his mother and two aunts sexually molested him.

Suddenly, I feel that my own life must now be revised, my own feelings, because not only do I hear his voice whispering his secret, I also imagine fleeting details of how it happened, and when. I imagine my father, that small boy in Russia, after his father left the family to move to America. My father is alone with his mother. His mother is frightened she'll never see her husband again, and so she turns, of course, to her son for comfort. And he will comfort her. He will do whatever is asked to stop his mother's weeping, to sponge up his mother's fear. And his mother? What had happened to her, what began the cycle, the long downward spiral, to me? They are Russian peasants. They live in long, dark Russian winters where a Czar's army stages pogroms to kill Jews. They live in an icy white wind that coalesces into a single brutal force. What comfort might my father's mother's father also have needed? My great-grandfather.

I imagine cold winter dust on the floor beneath the bed. I imagine mattresses, all of them stuffed with straw. I feel this mattress, yes, as if spears of straw are stuck in my own back. For they are. These are my roots. This is my inheritance. My legacy. My hope chest is filled with dry stalks of straw and tattered sheets. It is filled with pillows stuffed with fear. These hard, brittle mattresses are handed down from one generation to the next. Rage is handed down. Rage that we must sleep on straw mattresses during frigid Russian winters. So I imagine that my grandmother, my father, his grandfather must look for warmth and comfort elsewhere. And it is found. Found in the soft, scared body of a most malleable child.

I want to comfort my father now. I want to save him from the isolation of a Russian winter in a tiny shtetl outside Kiev. I want to save him from those nights. I see his arm thrust out from his body, reaching for air to hold onto, to pull him away from his mother. The air—cold, thin—won't support him. His gesture is futile. His mother's mouth will devour him. She is a creature with no soul. I imagine she suckles him for nourishment and sustenance, draining his soul from his body. And when she is finished, his aunts begin: one, then the other. I see him on a bed, his back speared by straw, pressed deeper and deeper into the mattress. The skin on his back bleeds. I imagine blood dripping onto frigid Russian soil.

My progress at the hospital stops. I can't get better. I can't get better as long as I want to save my father.

And I do.

Randy is angry my father has told me his secret. "He told you that to manipulate you," Randy says. "He told you so you won't blame him. He told you so you'd still love him. So you could excuse him for what he did to you."

"He told me because it's true," I say.

"But he shouldn't have told you. Not now. He doesn't want you to get better. He's scared about your getting better. He's scared you won't take care of his needs anymore. He's scared you're telling the family secret."

I know Randy is right. I suspect this *is* why my father told me. But the image of that boy in Russia lingers. It will linger forever. I imagine he's a boy who first lost his soul by the time he was three and could never reclaim it, because, with all the rage I know that lives in his body, I suspect his mother must have stolen his soul again and again, even as he grew older. *But, Daddy, I want to ask you, I want to know, did you think you'd reclaim your own soul by secretly stealing another?*

"Don't you see?" I say to Randy. "It had to happen. He had to do what he did to me because of his mother. He didn't have a choice. If that's what she taught him, that's the only thing he could have done to me."

Randy tells me my father was an adult when he molested me, adults have choices. He could have chosen to seek help. He could have committed himself to a hospital. He could have sent me to a place where I'd be safe. "You never molested anyone," he says to me. "Not everyone who's molested passes it on. What you do is keep hurting yourself."

□ □ □

Sunday is visiting day at the hospital. My husband won't arrive until afternoon, so I sit in the lounge in the unit where lamps are lit, warming the gray, rainy day, warming the room, as if this is a family living room and a small gathering of friends. I watch a woman named Macon, new in the unit, although she arrived here from the locked unit at Kennestone. This morning I sat next to her at breakfast where she showed me a round gash in her tongue resembling a cigarette burn. In fact, she'd convulsed on a drug overdose while trying to commit suicide and a tooth had sliced her tongue. Now, she silently stares at her hands folded in her lap, saying nothing to her family, looking down.

Her husband looks angry, his face thick with rage. Sweat spikes the dark hair on the nape of his neck and the hair looks as if it's bristling. I can't hear his words, but his gestures strike the air as he speaks. Their daughter—she must be in the third or fourth grade—sits on the floor with crayons and coloring book, her head bowed. Her hair is yanked into a messy off-center ponytail with clumps of hair spilling loose over her shoulders. Macon doesn't say a word; she remains silent, studying her hands.

Then I see it. My only surprise is that I didn't notice immediately. The daughter. Not just her hair is unkempt . . . For a moment I feel light-headed. I can't swallow. I feel as if I'm spiraling back in space, and can see back then—but also I am here. Now. The daughter wears her dress inside out. I lean closer to make sure. Yes, her back is to me and the label hangs outside the neck. Seams circle the shoulders, the waist, the sides, the hem. I *know* that either her father dressed her wrong in a hurry because he'd undressed her in a hurry or else she does this deliberately, wears her dress this way to send a message, a signal, telling her mother, in this most accurate language, she is having an emergency. But Macon refuses to see. Macon doesn't see what she sees, even took pills to ensure she'd never notice. She was willing to kill herself rather than know what she knows. But by sacrificing herself, she most truly was willing to sacrifice her daughter.

Without plan, I stand to move toward them. Even from here I feel the tight knot of their family, the bewildering combinations of relationships and roles of these three people, impossible to unravel. Macon's husband's gaze is a blank rage as he turns to me, drawing closer, as if he can't imagine how I could intrude on the rigid perimeter of his family—*his,* because I know that's how he sees it—that he's created. I can't enter this knot. I back away. All I can do is tell the therapists about Macon's daughter and hope they can save her if she needs it.

But what had I seen when I looked at Macon's daughter? I see a girl who is small, a girl who could never have seduced her father.

I see her. I also see another little girl, one who, in her own accurately mute language, showed her underpants at school, stopped going to school, broke her collarbone at daycamp when she, too, wanted someone to see she was having an emergency.

My husband sits on a vinyl chair in my hospital room while I'm propped on the bed, my knees up. He is tall, tan; he looks healthy and calm, which he must be to balance me, balance the fulcrum of our teetering marriage. He is telling me about teaching his classes, having dinner with friends, painting the guest bathroom. He urges me to get a job teaching when I leave the hospital. "If you spend more time with people, you'll feel better," he says. "Please, just don't go back to sitting alone in the house."

I nod my head and try to listen as he speaks of the exotic ordinary. I almost believe my husband throws me these sentences as a lifeline, hoping to reel me in away from my parents, reel me into our marriage, reel me into that which *is* blessedly ordinary: life. I believe I've failed at everything defined as "life," have disappointed him in every way. I'm a terrible cook. I barely clean the house. I'm scared to teach or to work. I'm scared to have sex with him. I won't have children with him, am terrified just at the thought of a baby growing inside my evil stomach. Even though I fail him, he doesn't leave me. Instead he encourages me, again and again, to absorb the ordinary. As much as I want to, sometimes I fear it's too late. I'm too far away to reach him.

The curtains in the room are open. Raindrops splatter the glass. Earlier I'd watched Macon's husband leave the hospital with their daughter. He'd walked quickly across the parking lot while his daughter, wearing a thin jacket, not a slicker, stumbled behind. And right now I'm not at all sure if I ever even want to be out there again, outside the hospital. Why would I want to live out there, when there are too many Macons and their husbands out there, too many childhood emergencies? Too many unsafe daughters.

"Quizzle misses you," my husband says.

Quizzle. Our new cat. Mack is smiling at me. Maybe his smile is slightly forced, but the fact he tries so hard to reach me is what devastates, is what makes me want to cry.

He tells me she howls more than usual when he gets home from work because she's lonely.

Quizzle. Before she crosses the Oriental rug in our living room, she pauses at its fringed border. She lowers her head and her eyes dart back and forth, inspecting the terrain. What scary figure lurks in the rug's design? Does Quizzle see a scorpion with raised tail or a coiled snake that she must sneak past? Slowly, her paws stepping gingerly, her head still low to the ground, investigating, she crosses the potentially dangerous expanse of carpet. I wonder if she'll ever trust the design in the rug not to harm her.

"Quizzle really wants you back."

I walk to Mack's chair. I kneel beside it. His hand is on the armrest and I place my forehead on it. For a moment his hand seems to stiffen, as if he's not sure what to do. We touch each other so rarely. I miss you, I miss you, I miss you, I whisper, too softly, I know, for him to hear. I don't know how to tell him this aloud. I'm scared of my feelings, scared I might truly love this man who loves me back. He, too, is silent. For different reasons we don't know this language of intimacy, don't know how to form or create the words of love. I know the language of seduction, the language of my father, the language of sex. The language of night. I want to say something different to Mack. But still I don't trust him, don't trust myself, don't trust feelings. Right now I am too sad to try.

□ □ □

One day in the hospital we're taken to a swimming pool. At first I refuse to go in the water. My body doesn't want to feel water; it doesn't want to feel anything. The staff encourages me to try, and I believe if I don't appear to get better they won't let me leave the unit. When I'm most sick, when my addiction is most strong, I can swim, go to parties, smile, socialize, be what appears to be normal. Now, when the addiction is receding, I feel like an invalid unable to function. *You are only feeling*—I hear Randy's voice in my head. So while in the pool I begin to cry. The water reminds me of bathwater, reminds me of the tub in Maryland, reminds me of my father touching me, reminds me of the rubber duck that watched us.

I swim to the side of the pool and press my forehead against the tiles. I'm angry at how much the world scares me, that I'm an adult who isn't capable of behaving as an adult. All I can do at the pool is cry because—I know—Randy's voice is always with me, telling me what I need to know—and I need to cry now because I couldn't cry the first time my father's hand touched me. But I don't think I'll ever get better. I don't think I have the will to feel every place on my body, every place he touched me. Or every time.

I believe this, even though years have passed since I left home, years have passed since he touched me. Whenever I returned to visit, didn't we act like a normal family? On many trips I brought a boyfriend. To protect myself? But no longer did I need protection.

And my boyfriends only saw the image presented—the myth—what we wanted them to see. I always tell my friends what great parents they are: During the sixties they supported college students who demonstrated against the war in Vietnam. My parents were involved in the civil rights movement from the beginning. They were liberal Democrats, while most of my friends' parents were conservatives. My friends envied me my parents, and so I treated my parents like parents, overwhelmingly pleased by my friends' envy. Sometimes, yes, my father held me, stroked me, hugged me too tight. But we didn't have sex again. It's as if we decided to remain friends after the affair had ended.

But why did he stop? Perhaps he's afraid I'll say "no" if he tries, or that I might tell someone, now that I'm older and no longer dependent on them. Perhaps he's no longer interested because I'm not a little girl. Perhaps he's outgrown the rage that drove his desire to rape. Or perhaps he's found another little girl to molest. Another little girl to rape.

□ □ □

All these years I have clung to my parents, clung to these people who stole my body from me, as if waiting for them to relinquish it. I want them to, not only for me, but for them. I must believe they are tormented by the discrepancy between what they surely wanted for their lives and the life they actually created—what they actually have. I want all of us to recover from the past. That my parents will die without having lived scares me. My sister scares me. She runs more than two hours a day, and I want her to stop. She still will not let herself get close to me. I still love her and want her to love me back. I want to know from what it is she's running. Is she, too, an Egyptian princess, fleeing? From what? While growing up I never considered the possibility that what my father did to me he did to her, too. I believed I was the only one, the chosen one. I had to believe he loved me more than he loved her. I had to believe that what he did to me *was* love, because it was the only love I had. Now—now I wonder. Did he try to molest her? Did my tough, brave sister know how to refuse?

□ □ □

In another phone conversation my father tells me he has seen a therapist and asks if I'll visit him when I get out of the hospital. "I want to talk to you," he says. He says he feels bad because he doesn't know me—and there isn't much time. Always, he wants me to visit; this is not new. Never has he said he feels bad because he doesn't know me; this is new. For a moment I feel the rage, and I almost say what I feel, but I can't. I can't say: *You don't know me because all you did was rape me.* But I say this: I tell him we don't know each other because we don't know how to talk to each other, and that even if I visit we still won't know how. I also tell him I'm afraid to visit. He doesn't ask why.

And I say this: I tell him that because his mother sexually molested him, that's how he interprets love.

This man, my father, does not slam down the phone in a rage. In his small, scared boy's voice he asks what I mean. I say he sexualizes love—that he doesn't know how to feel or give love unless it's sexual. It means he's scared of intimacy. "It means you're scared to let anyone know who you really are."

□ □ □

I was always scared to let anyone know who I really was, just as I was scared to know myself, scared to understand what happened to me. To protect me from this knowledge, I created Dina and Celeste. “They were part of your life-support system,” Randy says. As a child I needed their protection.

I’m grateful they helped me survive, even as now it is time to say good-bye, to understand they’re not truly real, that I’m the one in control, that I control them. The threads of their tenuous existence are interconnected with the addiction that dwells in a land of lies. If I can say the words “My father raped me,” if I can say the words “My mother let him,” then I no longer need to disperse my self into other beings. I don’t need to comfort myself with euphemisms; I don’t need to comfort myself with Dina’s silence; I don’t need to comfort myself with Celeste’s words of seduction; I don’t need to comfort myself with lies.

To Celeste and Dina these lies of course were truth, were *their* truths. But no longer can they be mine. In the hospital, as the addiction fades, Celeste and Dina fade—lies fade—as I learn the language of life. The longer I’m sober, the stronger I become, the weaker are Dina and Celeste. They seem to flow one into the other, becoming one before becoming nothing. Then my own glance is only mine. And I am finally me.

□ □ □

In the hospital I say to my mother, on the phone: “I was sexually molested when I was a child.”

“Your father.”

This is not a question, and I am unable to acknowledge or answer it.

“Oh, well,” she says, “I had a terrible childhood, too. People talk about things like this now, but back then, no one knew.”

“You knew,” I say. *She doesn’t see what she sees.*

"But I didn't understand," she says. "No one knew what it meant back then. How could I have left? How could I have supported two small girls?"

"Money?" I say.

"It's not like now, with women working. I asked my brother for five thousand dollars and he turned me down. What could I do? Patsy, Esey—everyone wanted me to stay with him. Everyone thought he was a wonderful husband."

"He would have had to pay you child support and alimony."

"When I was a child we were so poor. My father was an awful person. Cold. My mother was a saint, always singing, never complaining—with all us children to raise. I don't know how she did it."

I hang up the phone. I lie in bed enraged. Who are you, this person called mother, a mother who listened to her radio at night so she could pretend not to hear her husband rape her daughter? I don't know this mother who desired the status of wife and family more than she desired the safety of her daughters, more than she cared for our lives.

Later, Randy urges me to beat a pillow with my fists, pretending the pillow is my mother. I must do this, learn finally to turn rage outward, in a safe way, not inward on myself. I pretend, yes, this pillow is my mother—a mother who never guided me through childhood, never guided me into adulthood, into life. Later, I imagine the pillow is my father . . . *he's walking toward me, at night, entering my bedroom, lifting the sheet, entering my bed . . . No. You. Stop.* I raise my arm to stop him. My arm is strong, distinct, full of purpose and muscle and power. He will stop. If my mother won't protect me, I will protect myself. I beat the pillow harder. I do and I do and I do.

□ □ □

“What does your writing mean to you?” Randy asks. I’m leaving the unit in a few days and he’s worried. No longer will I have constant care. He wants me to learn to structure time in a way to keep myself safe. He wants me to continue writing as part of my recovery. “How did you start?”

“I began to write in 1976,” I say. “It’s like I *had* to.” I was married to my first husband, a lawyer involved with politics, who, like my father, leaves Washington with the Republicans in power, taking me with him. We move to a small coastal community he plans to develop—not by opening a bank—but through architectural preservation. Even though my first husband is kind, generous, decent, he’s emotionally distant. I don’t know how to love him any more than he knows how to love me. During the time we are together he never tells me he loves me. I tell him I love him, but I don’t know that word’s definition. I don’t understand marriage. I don’t understand how to be a wife. I am lost from the start because all I know is how to play a role, how to *look right*—what I learned from my parents. From them I learned the importance of appearances, not bothering with the inconvenience of a true inner life. So now I re-create the appearance of a normal middle-class family—while being unfaithful to my husband, while once again leading a double life.

After several years of this incomprehensible marriage, I begin to see a psychiatrist. Month after month I dutifully come to his office, yet I won’t / can’t / don’t talk about my parents, explaining there’s nothing to say about them. Nor do I talk much about my marriage and even less about my true self. Instead, I talk about sex; I talk about men. Men are sex. They're nothing more, nothing less. The clothes I wear to his office are short, low-cut. In these clothes, I tell this man about all the men with whom I've had sex. I want to impress him. Yet the more I talk about sex and engage in sex, the more I have a vague sense that something is very wrong. But I don't know how to tell this psychiatrist, or myself, what *is* wrong. I'm afraid to speak, afraid that all the words that matter, all the words I should be saying to this man, are the words I never learned, are the words my father never allowed. If I speak, I also believe I will be hurt—like the time my father taped my mouth shut when my sister left for college, when I wanted to tell him I was scared. My mouth doesn't know how to say what is true. It feels inanimate, exhausted with all my father's lies.

One day when he, too, perhaps is frustrated by my lack of progress, the psychiatrist asks me how I see myself. I almost open my mouth to speak. But then I don't, I can't, for I have nothing to say. How do I see myself? I see myself in these too-short shorts. I see myself in this too-revealing blouse. But surely this man seeks different information. I shrug and slouch in the chair. Since I don't know how I see myself, I have nothing to say.

He asks if I might like to try drawing a picture of myself and hands me a pad of paper and a pencil. I take them, even knowing I can't draw anything more complicated than a stick figure. I am unable to draw. I am unable to speak. Maybe I must begin at some ancient origin of language and draw petroglyphs. Maybe I must learn the hieroglyphics of the Egyptian princess. I feel as if I am primitive or mute. As a child I believed I *was* primitive and mute. I believed I understood the sounds and the scents of nature more clearly than the words of my family. I also created my own unspoken words—like those of my secret alphabet. I memorized languages of camouflage, the language of survival. If I speak the language of the tropics, I am the tropics. If I speak the language of New Jersey suburbs, I am everygirl of the New Jersey suburbs. Therefore, I am not me. As a child I wasn't taught the language of me. So I couldn't learn the language of me. I didn't even want to know I existed.

But now—how do I tell this psychiatrist, or myself, how I see myself? If I can't draw. If I can't speak.

Well, maybe I could try to write, I think. I've done a little writing. I've written college papers and articles on architectural preservation. Besides, I've always loved to read words, words other people have written. Certainly writing is easier than speaking. If I write, no one will hear me. If I write, I won't have to open my mouth. I wouldn't even have to show the psychiatrist or anyone else what I write, especially if it's no good. And besides, besides—even my *father* thought I was good enough to write his book.

On the way home I stop at a stationery store for paper. I set up a card table in the bedroom and place a portable Smith-Corona typewriter on top of it. I open up the ream of pale yellow paper, less expensive than white paper, since I'm not sure whether my words have any value. I roll a sheet of paper into the feeder and stare at it. I rest my fingertips on the keyboard. But how do I start? My fingers remain rigid, unable to type, as I realize, of course, that writing articles isn't exactly the same as writing about myself. It's as if I lack the secret key to unlock the rigid formation of the alphabet. I must rearrange the letters, shuffle them like a deck of cards. Gently, uncertainly, I press down the letter *I*. Slowly I begin to type, even though I'm not sure what I'm writing.

In fact I discover I know how to write only in that I don't know how to stop writing. I use the first ream of paper, then buy a second. I buy a third ream, have written over a thousand pages, before I even consider stopping—not at a true ending, but rather I finally allow words to drift into the margin and off the page. The book is not so much about me, though, as about a shadow of me. It's certainly not about me and my father. Even though I fill up more than a thousand pages, I try words tentatively, constructing a pathway of words I hope will lead me to me. Over the years, later, I discover it will take many more thousands of words, many more thousands of pieces of paper.

During this time my husband and I separate, are reunited. Separate again.

It is with this initial bundle of more than a thousand pages of paper, carefully placed in two stationery boxes, that I meet the man who will eventually become my second husband, a graduate student who teaches writing at a continuing education center at a local university. I decide I must know the worth of all these pages—whether I should bother retyping what I have written onto white bond paper. So I sign up for the class, even though I will have to ask a man I've never met before to read my more than a thousand pages of yellow paper. I'm scared he'll say no; I'm scared he'll say yes. Since I don't trust that my words themselves will be enough to convince him to read them, I slip into my short cut-off jeans and halter top for the first class. I carefully apply makeup and arrange my hair. I watch for him to take his seat in front of the class before I stroll past, wanting him to notice me, remember me, desire me—believing in the power of my body to be noticed, desired, remembered. More than I would ever trust my words or any sentence.

In class that first night I sit in the front row, my legs slightly parted, watching him, wanting him to watch me. Mack—his name is Mack—talks about irony, a word I've heard, but not a word I truly understand. He says irony is when the reader knows more than the protagonist, has a clearer understanding of events than the protagonist. He says irony is also when the punishment doesn't fit the crime. He says irony is when you say one thing but mean another. Irony is when things are not what they seem. I am about to stop listening. I am about to let this word "irony" drift into oblivion where it might take years before I discover it again.

But then I don't. I raise my hand and tell him, this instructor named Mack, I don't quite understand what he means. Will he explain it again? With patience, he does. I hear the definition again. I make a connection. I see our pretty houses and our pretty clothes, see our Fleetwood Cadillac, see all the people who admire my parents, see all the smiling family photographs—see this—almost connecting it with a vision of what is seen when the walls of the pretty houses implode, when the pretty clothes are stripped off bodies, when the images on the photographs are ripped off the paper.

Mack's smile is shy, not insistent. He agrees to read my unwieldly manuscript, carefully reaching for the two boxes, holding the boxes with hands that are gentle. His hands—they are as gentle, yes, as the hands of my Uncle Esey, a man who also loved words, who knew you must hold words carefully so as not to break or misuse them.

Yet I believe that Mack agrees to read my book only because of the way I dress, for surely he knows what I offer. Perhaps I think I must "pay" him with more than money.

But this isn't what he wants. He's not like the others. And although he has a patched-together definition of love himself at this time, still, months later, he says he loves me and wants to marry me. And maybe I marry Mack just because he does read my words—he is the first person to read them. It will be years, though, before I understand that what he really wants is to hear a stronger voice—not the shadowy, stuttered words, a mere scaffold of an uncompleted path of sentences that, even with the thousand pages, leads me forward with only the most tentative step.

I'm never able to tell the psychiatrist how I see myself. I'm never able to tell him about my parents.

It's only now, with Randy, I practice all the words I need to speak. I especially practice saying words that have always scared me. Over and over I chant the word "no," what I must learn to say to dangerous men. He has me repeat the phrase "thank you," what I want to say when complimented—a phrase I struggle with—since I've never believed I deserve praise or attention. I learn to ask for what I want. I learn to express what I need.

I think of other skills I have learned. I remember the time in seventh grade when a teacher commented that I had sloppy handwriting. Devastated by this criticism, I spent months practicing penmanship, copying pages out of books, until the teacher smiled approval. All I cared about then was the beauty of the handwriting, the perfection of the page, for I had nothing of my own to write, nothing of my own to say. But now, with Randy, I learn to speak, learn to write, the words of my own vocabulary.

□ □ □

On the hospital unit we meet for Spirituality Group. Today, with paper, crayons, ribbons, yarn, we are to give tangible form to our higher power, visualize it, create it. We must try to believe in a power greater than ourselves—a power, therefore, greater than our addictions. The way to recover from destructive behavior, addictive lives, is to discover spirituality.

Always, I'd thought I had none. But when the therapists say a higher power needn't be a god—can be anything, even nature—I think of my heart safely beating in stone, or of my body protected by hibiscus petals. Yes, by hiding in nature—in its language as well as in its strength and its beauty—I felt as if it guarded me, so that even if my father found my body I could pretend he didn't find me. A higher power. I think of my Christmas tree, of that night in New Jersey when I was protected by Christmas spirits. So now I reach for a pine-green piece of construction paper and a pair of scissors. Yes, that tree must have been spiritual. It was full of power far greater than my own.

Today, for my session with Randy, I have brought a photograph of myself to show him. It is the one taken in second grade, when I was ordered to hold the crayon in my right hand. Even with this misrepresentation, it is the photo, the image, I think of when I imagine the little girl.

The photo is in a cardboard cover. I open it and hand it to Randy, telling him the story of the crayon. He holds it carefully, softly exclaiming over the little girl like a proud parent.

Listening to Randy, I also begin to feel like a proud parent, and all I can do is beam.

"Why don't we 're-do' the photo," he says. "Hold a 'crayon' in your left hand. See how it feels." He places a pencil on the small coffee table in front of the couch where I'm sitting. "Let's pretend it's a crayon," he says. "What was your favorite color?"

"That dress was lime-green," I say. "I really loved that dress." I look at the pencil. "Okay. It's green."

"Would you like to pick it up?"

I reach for it with my left hand and hold it.

"How does it feel?" he asks.

Quickly, in my mind, I run through the list of feelings Randy has taught me: mad, sad, glad, scared. "Glad?" I say.

He nods. "Anything else?"

I run the pencil across my fingers. I hold it as if about to write, then grip it tight in my fist. For a moment the pencil almost feels as strong as a magic wand. I glance back at Randy and say, "Powerful."

Now it is his turn to beam.

He puts the photograph on the coffee table, face up. We both look at her. She smiles straight into the camera. Yes, she—*I*—would never have let anyone know I was angry that the crayon had been taken from my left hand. Nor would I have let anyone know I was angry that my mother and father weren't with me to ensure I be allowed to hold the crayon properly. Later, when I'd explained to my mother what had happened, she'd told me not to worry about it, it was only a photograph. It doesn't mean anything, she'd said. It doesn't matter.

I reach over and lightly touch the face in the photo. I look at her eyes. I want to reach her. I want to touch her. I want to hold her hand. I want to wash her, dress her, feed her, love her. I want to whisper to her . . . I want to say to her, I *do* say: It does matter. *You* matter.

"But who loved her?" I whisper to Randy. "Loved me? Didn't my parents? My father always told me he loved me."

"They did love you," Randy says. He straightens and leans toward me as if hoping I'll feel his words, feel the power of his words, more strongly if they travel a shorter distance. "But their kind of love was hurtful and destructive. Little girls shouldn't have to be scared of their parents' love."

We are silent. Randy has tears in his eyes, yet he doesn't turn from me or wipe them away. I am confused. I don't understand who this man is or what this means. But—no—this time I will not be confused. This time I will let myself see him, will not turn away from him either. I allow myself to understand that *their* kind of love is not *his* kind of love, his, which isn't hurtful or destructive. I want to understand the foreignness of this man, a man who knows how to love well. His generosity, his love, his safety, his wisdom, his patience are almost too much. Yet this moment I allow his steadfast heart to warm my own once-dead heart. It is this, allowing myself to accept Randy, that will heal me.

"But suppose *I* never learn how to love the way *you* know how to love," I say.

"You *do* know how."

"But I don't feel like I do."

"Look at how you've cared for friends," he says. "Look at the men you've most cared about."

Christopher. Mack. "*You,*" I say. "I care about you."

"I know that," he says, smiling. "Otherwise you wouldn't keep coming back here week after week." He pauses and nods toward the photo. "And, most important, you care about her."

It is time to leave the hospital. I go home with my Christmas tree cutout. I go home with the pencil gripped tight in my left hand. I go home understanding that the girl's smile in the photo is not a smile that seduced my father. It is just a little-girl smile—both special and ordinary—a little girl, who I always wanted to be.

Two Small Rooms in Minnesota

In the mid-1980s my parents move to Rochester, Minnesota. To me, it seems as if they go there to die, although to live in a retirement complex associated with the Mayo Clinic is not without logic. This move scares me. I don't want to feel my fear of their deaths, so I look for the joke. I tell my friends I have the only parents in the world to retire in frigid Minnesota. Visiting them in Minnesota is scary. Who are these two old people? Have I ever known anything about them? They're going to die with all their secrets intact. They're going to die alone, even as they're surrounded by people. I want to imagine they have souls that will slip from their mouths as they exhale their last breaths.

In the restaurant on the top floor of the retirement complex, my parents' friends meet me. They exclaim about my wonderful parents. I smile and agree. What a fascinating career my father has had, they say. I smile and agree. My father gives lectures wowing people with the breadth of his knowledge. After one of his lectures a letter to the editor appears in the local newspaper with the headline "Positively Electrifying." The letter ends by saying, "Dr. Silverman, those who know you must truly love you!"

I want to bolt. Because of the hypocrisy? Because my parents have gotten away with it? There is no one to significantly disturb their final days, interfere with their decorum. Even if I told these people in the restaurant the truth about my parents, they would not hear me. The truth would be too difficult to consider. After all, each table is set with linen and flowers. The arrangement is too pretty. Who would want to disturb it? Who would want his or her equilibrium interrupted? No one wants to hear; so no one will know. But of course *I* am the one who says nothing, who can't tell these people, who can't confront my parents. So maybe I—not these people, not my parents—really, I am the one unable to face it.

Instead, like a Fundamentalist preacher, I am obsessive in my mission to "save" them before they die, as if *I* can be the one to nourish their souls. I talk about spirituality, about the need to discover a higher power, to believe in something greater than ourselves. I ask my parents about themselves as children. Mom—what were you really like as a child? Dad—who were you? I want them to remember themselves, *find* something within themselves that's gentle. Surely they—all of us—began as sweet, cute children. Or maybe I am the one who wants to know them as children. Before they die, I want to be able to love them, if not as adults, then as children, as who they were when they were little. But even though they listen to me, they don't understand me and aren't able to respond to anything I say.

In a way, though, perhaps *they* help to "save" me instead, by giving me what they always provide: money. When my insurance ends they agree to pay for my therapy. And while money isn't spiritual, it helps, is a way they can help "save" me, even as they don't understand that what happened in the past is why I need it.

□ □ □

While visiting them I sleep in a blue sweatshirt with an emblem of Mickey and Minnie Mouse across the chest. One evening when I'm saying good-night to my mother, she reaches forward to touch it, pretending she wants to see the design more clearly. I step back. She steps forward, her arm still outstretched. Unable to say "stop," I again step back until I'm against the wall. She laughs awkwardly, asking what's wrong. I say the word "boundaries." She doesn't understand. I draw an imaginary line in front of my body. Still she doesn't understand I now own my body and she can't touch it. In her need she lunges forward—I try to turn—but her fingertips graze my chest.

My father has diabetes, and in the morning the resident nurse comes to check his blood sugar. My father is in his underwear, but I don't want the nurse to see him this way or know this is the way we live. Since I'm afraid to say anything to him, I whisper to my mother, "I think it'd be better if he put on a robe." She doesn't say anything to him either, but she hands him his robe. He puts it on but then fails to tie it.

□ □ □

Shortly after they move to Minnesota my father undergoes heart surgery. I fly up immediately; my sister doesn't follow. My mother catches a cold and can't visit him in the hospital, so I am the one to stay with him for hours, days, alone with him—my duty. Am I a martyr? I believe my impulse is fear: If I don't do what is expected my parents won't love me. I, the adult, am still not able to love her, the child, enough by myself.

As my father recovers he kisses the nurses' hands and flirts with them—this sick old man who is dying. He must tell every nurse on every shift about his career to ensure they know how lucky they are to be allowed to care for him. He believes he has graced the hospital with his presence. I want to scream, *Daddy, nobody cares.* I say nothing. I sit in the plastic chair in his hospital room and stare out the window at a bitter winter sky. To me, he will describe in detail the bath the nurse gave him earlier this morning. Now, he says, he feels clean all over. Is this an invitation? Again I say nothing. My father will never stop. I know I will never have the power to stop him.

Soon after the operation my father's mind begins to slip into other realities, even though, to him, little has ever been real. To hide my fear, I joke to Randy that my father has "slipped his gears." This is how I see it, though. His mind, once knobby with information, spins smooth, grooveless, as he chucks out unneeded and unwanted facts. He creates a fantasy fourteen million dollars that my sister and I are to inherit and presses me to set up a company to handle the money. Have I hired a lawyer? he asks. For weeks he grills me about plans for the corporation. He wants the board of directors to meet with him. I do not try to reel him back to reality. As I have always done, I enact the play with him, play the role I am assigned by him, and allow his mind to float far away from the inconvenient confines of his skull. When my patience thins and I barely respond he gets angry—and still the little girl gets scared.

Finally, in the middle of the night he sneaks from their apartment and is found wandering outside. He must be moved from their apartment down to the third floor of the complex, a nursing unit, where he receives constant care.

Even though she never smoked, my mother gets lung cancer and needs surgery. When the surgeon calls to say the operation was a success, my feelings are ambiguous. I'm not truly relieved; yet, while I knew the operation was being performed, I compulsively cleaned my house.

While my father is on the third floor of the complex, my mother now moves to the fourth, where the residents' problems are physical. They will never return to their apartment, never again be together. During the past few months, my sister and I have spoken more frequently then ever before, not just dividing up our parents' possessions, but also, perhaps, needing to hear each other's fear as our parents die. Now, over Christmas, I fly to Rochester to ready their things for the movers.

I am alone in my parents' apartment. Outside their twelfth-floor window is a gray December day. Inside, I am awed by silence. My parents will never be in these rooms again, will never see their lifetime collection of furniture, paintings, art objects, photographs, books. They will never eat from their plates or drink from their glasses. They will never use their silverware. These objects seem still and waiting, as if willing to accept the inevitability of a thin layer of dust until they have been relocated, willing to accept the inevitability of a new location. These objects owned by my parents will outlive my parents, yet their footsteps will always be felt in the weave of rugs, the touch of their fingers felt on the skin of glass vases.

The apartment is not large—two bedrooms. Still, I wander in and out of the rooms. I open closets and stare at shoes and clothes. Pink sandals. L. L. Bean boots. Some clothes still have tags. For my parents the end has come suddenly, now that it's finally come. In the pantry is a file cabinet filled with business papers and personal letters, saved over the years. My sister wants to throw all the letters away, but I will save everything. In the refrigerator is a half-finished loaf of rye bread. Fruit-juice bottles not yet empty. *Daddy. Mom. I want you to be able to finish them.*

I touch their possessions as if I have never before seen them. There are vases, plates, and tea sets that my father bought in Occupied Japan after the war. There are masks and fans from the South Pacific islands. A set of Wedgwood plates from the West Indies. Candlesticks my parents purchased in Israel, when it was still Palestine. Oriental rugs from the Middle East. A handwoven rug from South America. Antique photograph albums. Silks from Hong Kong. An enameled plate from Egypt. Engraved plates from Puerto Rico. Furniture my father built, years ago, with that electric saw. There are bits and pieces of households from Washington, Maryland, St. Thomas, and New Jersey.

My father's bedroom is a shrine. Every morning, upon waking, he was able to worship himself, worship his success. The walls are crammed with signed photographs of governors, senators, congressmen. There is a photo of Justice Louis Brandeis, since my father prepared the legal brief on behalf of the United States Government in the Edwards (*The Grapes of Wrath*) case, argued before the Supreme Court. A letter from President Truman, framed with a photograph and a presidential pen, commends my father's work on behalf of Guam. There are pictures of bank openings. A photo of my father with his colleagues on the Hackensack Meadowlands Development Commission. And more. Most of these men are dead, of course. Of those still living, none will be with my father as he dies. None will call. Relationships remain lifeless photographs. But tucked among the mementos, hung on the wall close to his pillow, is that one small photo of our family at the opening of the Saddle Brook Bank. My father stands between my mother and me—my sister slightly detached. My father beams. How proud he is of the lovely picture he created.

In the closet I find my mother's button jar and pour all the buttons onto the rug. I trail my fingers through them, inspecting each one. Blue buttons, red buttons, white buttons. Leather buttons, metallic buttons, glass buttons. Plain plastic buttons. Buttons with intricate designs. Buttons with thread still dangling from the holes. Buttons covered with material. A pearl button with a fake diamond center. All these buttons managed to survive all the shirts, skirts, slacks, sweaters, shorts, all the clothes worn by my family.

One special button I put in my wallet to carry home with me on the plane. It is a white button with two large holes for eyes. Around the holes, eyebrows and eyelashes are painted. Below, in red paint, is a dot of a mouth. A button face. A yellow playsuit with button-face buttons. Perhaps the playsuit had first been my sister's, then mine. I see them: all our playsuits, all our pretty cotton dresses, our pinafores, our jumpers, our sailorsuit dresses, all swaying on a clothesline in a summer breeze. I imagine I lie on the grass and gaze up at our playsuits, at our dresses, almost transparent in blinding white sunlight. I see this thinness of material, like a transparency of an undeveloped photograph, with no little-girl bodies inside.

At the bottom of a wooden trunk, under a pile of blankets, I find my senior high school yearbook. I haven't seen it in years, and had lost track of my high school friends shortly after graduation. I sit on the floor and skim the pages of photographs, a chronicle of proms, class plays, sporting events. I turn to the senior class pictures. Jane—still smiling her New Jersey smile, one I never learned to imitate. Christopher. His young, innocent shyness is frozen in time, his face one I will never forget. I lean close to read the faded inscription, wanting to recall what he thought to write to me years ago.

"Dear Sue—What I say now I mean sincerely. You have been a part of my life that I will never forget. I'll remember the good times, the bad times, and the confusing times. Love, Christopher."

I wonder if he does still remember those times. *Christopher, do you remember me as often as I remember you?*

I turn to my own picture. I stare straight into the camera. My hair, the flip I adored, is still rigid, sleek, perfect.

I close the yearbook and ruffle my long curly hair. No longer do I need to look perfect.

In my father's desk I discover a leather journal. Embossed in gold on the cover are the words "My Trip Abroad." It is a honeymoon journal kept by my father when he and my mother sailed to Palestine. Inside is a dried red rose pressed into the cover with a short item from an October 27, 1933, Chicago newspaper:

CHICAGO ATTORNEY AND BRIDE PLAN
TO LIVE IN PALESTINE

> Irwin Silverman, young Chicago attorney, and Fay Silverman, who are to be married Sunday in the home of the bride's parents, Mr. and Mrs. M. Silverman, 515 S. Central Ave., plan to make their home in Palestine. Immediately after the wedding they will leave for a honeymoon in Ireland, France, Italy, Switzerland, Greece, Turkey, Smyrna and Egypt. From

there they will go to Palestine, where Silverman plans to join a firm of attorneys.

They sailed on the M.V. *Georgic* of the Cunard White Star Line on Friday, November 3, 1933, at 8:45 P.M., from New York City. The captain was F. F. Summers. I want to hold time in my hands, contain it. I want this trip back. I want the clock to read 8:44, and they have one last minute before sailing. They have just been married. But this time, before the ship sails, in this final minute, but a long-long minute, the ship must be delayed while a squall batters the harbor. All the leaves gust from trees, all the feathers fall from wings of the birds, and in this violence of nature, *they*, my parents, must balance nature. They must be the calm. So this time when the ship sails, the journey will be different. They will not return on the M.V. *Brittanic*, September 15, 1935, two years later. Maybe if they'd never returned to the States, maybe if they'd stayed overseas, then they would have been different.

I remove the rose from the journal. It smells of ancient, dusty paper and crushed burgundy petals. I am awed it has survived the years. I imagine my father purchasing it for my mother the morning they married. What was he thinking that morning? Who was he that morning? Would he even once remember his mother, his first years in Russia? Surely his parents and brother and sisters would be at the wedding, even though his mother vehemently objected to the match. She insisted that my mother was beneath her son, that her truly beloved son could do better.

My parents had met on a beach, introduced by my father's cousin, who also knew my mother. By chance they had the same last name because immigration officials redefined their parents' identities by baptizing each family "Silverman." I want to ask my parents if part of the attraction between them was a narcissistic whiff of incest: We are the same name; you are me; and I am only capable of loving my own image.

On their first date my father proposed marriage, although my mother initially refused. For weeks he persisted, threatening suicide if she didn't acquiesce—until she did. What was his persistence, his obsession, his compulsion, his need? *Did you know I was coming, Daddy, a baby girl just for you?*

I replace the rose inside my father's honeymoon journal. Most truly, it can only smell bitter.

Now, my mother is alone in her room, my father alone in his. They do not see each other, for my mother refuses to see him. Enraged, my father tries to escape to find her, hissing to me that the Nazis have kidnapped him and won't allow him to return to his apartment. Later, he will sob that my mother has left him. The nurses secure an anklet on him that sounds an alarm when he crosses the third-floor boundary. Finally a boundary is established for him—his first ever. He is contained, trapped. He can't reach any of his three little girls. And all it takes, *all* it takes, I see now, is a thin plastic band around his ankle, a band to sound an alarm. If only I had known this—how simple.

My mother sees him only one more time. After she learns the cancer has spread to her other lung, she goes to his room once to say good-bye. She will cry. He will not fully understand what is happening, only understand it is bad. I want to comfort him. I want . . . No longer do I even know what I want. Just not this. I don't want my parents to die, each alone, in separate rooms. I want to bring them home with me. I want to baptize them with balms to cool fevers. I want to give them life. Over and over, like a mantra, I tell my father I love him. He tells me the same thing back. These words he remembers. But still I doubt if he understands what the word "love" means.

As I sort through my parents' possessions, it's difficult for me to part with anything because there wasn't enough love in our family. In the same way I have gorged on sugar, I now try to stuff myself full of my parents' trinkets as if, by the weight of these objects alone, I will feel weighted with love. The cost of the items isn't the issue. If my parents were homeless I would fill a plastic garbage bag with every scrap of tattered rag. If my parents had fifty cents I would hoard my quarter, resigned that I had to give my sister the other half. In a pocket of my father's sports jacket I discover a package of Lifesavers. I sit on the floor of the hallway gripping it, knowing I will never part with it. I am almost overcome with the image of my father walking into a drugstore and buying it, making the selection. Why this package of five flavors and not another? Cherry, lemon, lime, strawberry, orange. The package is unopened. Surely this is one of the last things he purchased. He never had the chance to place one on his tongue to let it dissolve, allowing him to concentrate on the flavor for a few moments rather than concentrate on—what? This package of Lifesavers I put in my suitcase with his honeymoon journal; I wouldn't want the movers to accidentally lose it. When I get home I put it in a drawer with my jewelry.

I decorate my father's room with photographs of his family—his family of origin and also us, the family he created. I put a pretty plaid blanket on his bed. In his closet I stuff too many of his clothes from the apartment, even a sports jacket and tie, as if his condition is temporary. It isn't. A series of small strokes causes my father's dementia. His circulation has slowed, almost stopped, causing his hands and feet to swell until the skin cracks.

But even with his dementia—no, because of it—I can talk to him now, as if for the first time. His mask is gone. His career is gone. The face he wears in the world is lost to his dementia, and now he is alone with himself. He's not in time or space as we know it, but does that matter? Sometimes he believes I'm his sister, sometimes his daughter, but it doesn't matter. He is quiet, almost gentle.

He tells me his mother and father should never have married, that his mother used to beat his father with a stick, beat him with a stick. His mother was cruel, he says. She hurt him. Even though he is over eighty now, I see the hurt little boy in his eyes, in his face. And I have to ask him what she did to him, even though I understand it's not right for me to know. "How did she molest you?" I whisper, bending close to him, our eyes level. His hand makes a small gesture toward his face. "With the mouth," he whispers back, our secret. "My mother was a whore." This is all he says about it.

"Your mother and I should never have married either," he says. And because the room is stuffy, because his skin is cracked and dry, because he is always asking for glasses of water, he says, with an odd accuracy of a mixed metaphor, "She and I were like glass and water." His smile is small, almost timid. "You and I are exactly alike."

I wonder what part of him says this. Is it the father of my childhood or the father who's now dying? I wonder if he remembers us, the way we used to be. I wonder if this is why he loved me the way he did. *You and I are exactly alike*. Incest. In his narcissism he could only love his own image. He'd even given me the same middle name as his own, which was also his father's name: William. He didn't love me, could never have loved me. He could only love himself.

Later that same evening, after this conversation about his mother, his mind worsens as if quickly needing a strong fix of the soothing drug dementia. Every fragment of his mind seems to disperse, profoundly forgetting secrets lived, secrets revealed. He is restless. Trying to leave his wheelchair, he falls. The nurses put him in bed but he tries to get out. Again he falls. When they place restraints on him he thrashes his arms and screams, terrified. He has never worn a seat belt, always got angry when asked to wear one, has always been claustrophobic. Now, I know why: He is a young boy. He is pinned to a bed of straw. His limbs feel paralyzed. And so they are.

Tonight neither the nurses nor I can calm him. I try giving him juice. I show him pictures of the family. I talk to him, but he waves me aside. I ask him if he knows who I am.

"Of course I know who you are." His voice is angry.

"Who?"

"Josephine Missouri."

No one. Anyone. A meaningless name. A random selection of words pieced together in the jumble of a mind disassembling. Josephine Missouri. Maybe to him I always was—and am. Later, when I tell Randy what he called me, I am almost able to smile.

My mother wants no photos of the family in her room. No mementos of her life. No flowers. No decorations. She slips off her wedding ring and gives it to me. She hands me the money in her wallet. All she's brought with her from her apartment is her radio, her closest companion. She will be listening to news or a talk show on politics, I know, when she dies. World leaders, political leaders, the state of Israel—distant voices on a radio, faraway events and places—are her closest friends. Even disasters, like wars in the Middle East, comfort her, actually suit her better, since disasters create more of a distraction, consume more energy, more time. *Oh, Mother,* I want to say to her, *why don't you feel sad because you struggled to love your family, because you struggled to love your life?*

I know I never fully understood her life. On the counter in her bathroom in their apartment is a small cut-crystal vase filled with miniature dried flowers. Surrounding it is a girlish arrangement of perfume. Most of the perfume is from St. Thomas, yet the seals have never been broken. She has saved this perfume all these years as if for an emergency. I realize I never knew the girl (I must call her a girl, here), who arranged this girlish display. I never knew the girl who waited for a stranger good enough for her to sample her perfume. Who—what did my mother want? Did she desire me or my father? Did she want us to stop or desire for us to continue while she waited for someone worthy of her perfume? Did she want to preserve our family, our home? Did she want us all to fall apart?

I sit with my mother in her room as she drifts into sleep. I switch off her radio and lean back in the chair, watching her. It is dusk. Just before dinner. A wedge of light from the hall seeps into the room. Her breath is faint, her sleeping body still. In this absence of sound, in this quiet, quiet light, I wonder if she senses me here, close to her. *Mom, do you know your daughter is with you, waiting for you to waken? Do you know this is what daughters are meant to do, be with their mothers while their mothers are dying, be with them because they want to?*

Now, as she is dying, I wonder if she remembers those moments, those times, when I must believe she *did* want to preserve our family, when she wanted us to *be* a family, when she understood what she must do as a mother, when she understood the definition of the word "daughter." I want to ask her if she remembers—I want to ask her if she knows who was the mother I called that one particular night, years ago, the mother who knew how to listen, the mother who knew how to whisper the word "sorry," the mother who wasn't scared?

It was the time, it was one night, when I was in my early twenties, Mother. It was night, late at night. All evening I'd sat on the black corduroy couch in my apartment, the telephone on my lap. All night the night felt as if it would last as long as my life, as if it would never ease forward. I hadn't moved all night, had continued to hold the phone after he'd called to say he didn't want to see me again. All I could imagine for the rest of the night, for the rest of my life, were men falling both toward me and away from me like dominoes. So I gripped the phone as if it were all that remained of the relationship. It was all that remained of any relationship. I didn't know how to release the phone. I was afraid to. I was afraid to go to bed. I believed I had to hear something, know something, feel something, before I'd be able to release the phone and go to bed. I believed, at that moment, I needed to hear my mother.

"What is it, dear?" she'd said when she answered the phone. "What time is it? Is something wrong?"

"I think I'm kind of having an emergency."

Of course I had awakened her. I imagined her fingers clutching the buttons of her bathrobe. I believed I said the word "emergency" to be sure she'd hear me, a news flash on her radio, and that even now she was imagining a fire, a car wreck, cancer, three weeks to live, or random violence, paralyzed from the neck down.

But I also said the word "emergency" because right before I called I'd heard a siren splitting the night, sure it raced toward me to rescue me, here, where I sat on the black corduroy couch in my living room all night, having an emergency.

"Tell me," she urged. "What's wrong."

"It's just—" Now I wasn't sure how to describe the melodrama of an emergency.

"Did something happen? You need money?"

"No, no. I don't need money. I need—"

You.

"I don't know," I said. "I mean, maybe if you're not too tired we could just—" *I'm all alone, Mom, help me. Please just don't hang up the phone.* "Maybe talk a little while."

"Of course we can talk, dear. But tell me what happened. A man?"

"Well, kind of." I wanted to speak; I was scared to speak. I leaned back against the couch and pressed the palm of my hand against my mouth. I felt pressure, where it always began, in my throat, rising hard toward my mouth. This pressure scared me. I was scared it might leak out. Once it started leaking . . . I curled my fingers into a fist and pressed my knuckles against my neck. "It's just, things don't seem to be working out the way I want them," I said.

"Yes, yes, I understand, dear. They never do."

"But I mean *really*."

"I had no idea," she said. "Don't worry. One day you'll meet the right man. I promise."

The pressure deepened. I pressed my knuckles harder. "But maybe I'm not the 'right' girl."

"Why you're a lovely girl. You're friendly. Intelligent. Any man—"

"Mother. Wait. I think I'm really, really—not doing too well," I said.

For a moment there was silence. The siren had faded. Our voices had faded. Then, very softly, she said, "Oh, dear. I'm so sorry."

Slowly I released my fist from my throat. *Sorry,* I'd whispered to myself. *Sorry.* A word I'd waited to hear, a word to ease me through the night, a word to protect me until morning.

Now, as my mother is dying, I wonder if maybe *I* am the one who needs to remember those moments, those times, remember there are other words to hear, other voices that must be remembered.

□ □ □

In March, when I return to Minnesota, my father's face has yellowed. His cheeks are sunken, pulling his lips back to expose his teeth. His eyes are dim, the skin across them gluey. Sores and scabs cover his feet and hands. His ears brown in decay. Whoever he once was seems lost to sulphuric clouds of a futuristic landscape inhabited by skeletal creatures in a place unable to sustain skin, organs, blood, life. Still, when he sees me, for this moment, now, the expression on his face seems to rise from his polluted landscape and glow with joy. This lasts only a moment. I want to hold it—and can, and do—in my mind.

This visit he can barely speak, and I can barely understand him. He sleeps more. But every time he opens his eyes I tell him I love him. He nods his head and mouths, "I love you, too." I want more. I say these words insistently, as if now, even at this late moment, he can be redeemed, as if something can be said or done, if not to erase the past, then to diminish it. If he would ask forgiveness. If he would tell me he'd made a terrible, terrible mistake. If he would even just acknowledge it. But the past, in an inversion of time, seems to have fled to that futuristic landscape choked with sulphuric clouds. Still, like a stubborn, willful, yet loving child, I sit by him in his room, waiting for some acknowledgment before he dies.

Later, I leave his room and go to sit with my mother in hers. This trip I seem to journey back and forth between my father's room on the third floor and my mother's room on the fourth, as if I hope to discover a new answer to the mystery at the end of this incomprehensible voyage. Or perhaps I can entreat new spirits to invade my parents' bodies, quickly, before they die. To help me, I want to light candles, inhale incense, perform a secret ceremony. Now I gaze into my mother's eyes as I'd gazed into my father's, as if searching for someone new, searching for clues. Except in their eyes I see no new spirits, no new clues. And still I do not see eyes that reflect their daughter.

If only I could hear, once again, the mother and daughter who spoke on the phone that night, now, before she dies. If only my mother and I could discover a way to say good-bye to each other, if not with truth, then at least with grace. We cannot. For ceaselessly, during recent phone calls, she has demanded to know whether I would, if I could, provide her with enough pills to kill herself, even though she knows legally I can't. "This would be an act of love," she says, her voice brittle as glass, announcing Kiki would do it for her. What she wants to know is: Do I love her as much as Kiki loves her, love her enough to kill her? What I want to ask her, what I want to know, is whether this is an inverted test of her daughters' love or whether her desire is darker, an ancient ritual she needs performed. But how can she not know that even if I magically conjured the sleeping pills she desires, there would never be enough tablets, potions, or incantations to truly ease her journey?

"Can I bring you a tray, Mom?" I ask her, since it's almost time for dinner.

"This's plenty." In a small plastic baggie my mother keeps a meager supply of nuts—breakfast, lunch, and dinner. Now, with a thin hand she reaches into the bag for an almond, then slides it slowly, lovingly, into her mouth as if believing this one nut will summon starvation rather than prolong life.

"How about juice?"

"No. Nothing."

I can understand a desire to die because she's in pain. What I don't understand is her desire to die coldly, to die without comfort, die in isolation. Now, I wonder, I wonder if it's possible, I wonder if she decided to die that moment I told her, when I was in the hospital, that I'd been sexually molested. At that time I thought she'd barely heard what I said. She'd barely responded to what I'd said. But maybe, overwhelmingly terrified to acknowledge her fear behind the truth of our family, *this* is her response: Unable to protect her daughters, she thinks she deserves to die. I think of Macon, that woman who'd tried to kill herself, because she, too, was scared to see and to hear her daughter. Couldn't Macon have found another way? Can't my mother, can't we, can't all of us, find another way, discover something better, something softer, than dying alone in small rooms of fury and shame? *Oh, Mother, how can you not know that a simple apology would do?*

"Maybe I could just stay with you while you eat." I nod toward her nuts.

"I'm fine." Slowly my mother crunches her one thin almond. "Go eat with your father. You know how happy he always is to see you."

As I obediently stand to retrace my steps back downstairs to my father, I pause by the door and glance back. *Mother, a simple desire for you to want to eat with me, for you to always be happy to see me, would be enough, would do.*

I eat dinner with my father in order to feed him. He needs help eating. With the swelling in his hands he can't manage silverware. I cut his food and hold it to his mouth, small bite after slow bite. We sit with the other patients, all in various stages of sanity and life. Music from the 1940s tries to calm the inhuman sounds of dementia. Yet I am tense, as if tenseness can protect me from the sounds of dying, protect me from where all of us are eventually going. When I call my husband, he says when we baby boomers hit the nursing homes they'll play rock music and give us tie-dyed bibs to catch our drool. I imagine tapping a gnarled finger to the Beatles and the Rolling Stones.

So, yes, I feed my father. I hold apple juice and coffee to his lips. I cut his banana and his meat. Like a recalcitrant child, he won't eat his vegetables. His eye is on the ice cream, and he wants to eat it first, he wants to eat it *now*, before his dinner. Why not? Since I eat with him, I eat my ice cream first, too. We smile at each other, two naughty children—always—breaking the rules.

Late at night, unable to sleep, I call Randy's office, only needing to hear his answering machine and leave a message. I tell Randy about feeding my father. In my mind I hear him answer: *You've always fed your father.* I would nod my head, agreeing. *Would you like to stop?* he would ask. Yes, I want to stop. Being here, feeding my father, I feel as if I've never stopped. *You can stop feeding him,* Randy, I imagine, would say. *He can't hurt you any longer if you stop.*

But I'm scared to stop feeding him. I feed him because I love him, because I can't stop loving him. I feed him because I can't stop wanting him to love me. I feed him because he needs it so badly, feed him because he's never been nourished. I feed him and feed him—just one more time, I tell myself. I'll feed him one more time and this time, this will be the time, when everything will turn out different, this will be the time I'll have the family I always wanted.

I hug my mother good-bye, hug her, I know, for the last time. The skin on her shoulders is a loose fit for her frail bones, yes, rejecting her body as quickly as possible. Yet I hold her shoulders tight, as if I can hold her together, as if I can insist she feel me, feel the warmth of her daughter now, before she dies. "Mom." *Don't leave yet. I'm not ready.* Perhaps if I remind her of that late-night phone conversation—perhaps if she hears and remembers her daughter's voice, she'll want to live. "Mom," I whisper. "Wait, remember—"

"You have such a kind husband," she says. "And your therapist—"

"Yes, I know, I'm very lucky."

"After we're gone you'll have enough money. You won't need to worry."

"Yes, I know, thank you. But, *Mom*—"

She sighs and shrugs her shoulders. No, I can't remind her of that phone call. I'm scared to remind her, scared she won't remember. Slowly I release her shoulders, my mother's shoulders, my mother, the antithesis of my father, my father who needs too much, while my mother needs too little, rejecting nourishment and care, even now as she's dying. Still she's terrified to allow her family to warm her, much more terrified of this than of dying. Slowly, I back out of the room. She seems to be dissolving. White hair. White skin. White sheets. Her blue eyes are her only color. They aren't bright or sparkling but are deeper, bluer than usual, as if all that she is has coalesced to these blue eyes. I pause in the doorway, gently letting my own eyes say good-bye, letting my eyes say, *wanting* to say . . . It is too late. There is no more time. *But, Mom—all I ever wanted was you.*

□ □ □

Two weeks later, on Friday, April 3, 1992, the phone call comes: My mother is dead. The nurse who calls says that after my mother died the rabbi brought my father into my mother's room to say good-bye. "Do you think he understood?" I ask. "It's difficult to know, but probably," she says. I imagine the scene the nurse describes. My father is hunched in his wheelchair. He takes his wife's hand and holds it, this last time. His wife. After all these years, this is virtually the first time he's seen her in months. He will stroke the papery skin on her hand, the raised vein that travels between her knuckles. What will his heart want to tell her that's too late for his voice to say? *But Daddy, you always told me she never heard anyway.* The nurse says he motioned for her, the nurse, to bend down, and she imagined he'd wanted to tell her something. He kissed her cheek instead. He probably thought I was you, she says to me, and I agree. For weeks I believe this. And maybe it's true. But I think of the nurses he kissed in the hospital, and I believe it could have been anyone.

My husband and I take the next plane to Rochester. *I'm coming, Father, for you.* Since he knows my mother is dead, I want him to know there will still be someone to care for him. *I'm coming,*

Father, for you. He must know this; he must feel the plane drawing closer and closer. I literally can't stand the thought he'll believe he's alone. Right now nothing that happened matters. I have to be with him, that's all.

By the time we reach my father's room he's sleeping. My husband and I stand by his bed gazing down at him. He's curled like a sick, feverish child, and I bend to touch his forehead. He is small, helpless, innocent. He is vulnerable. Unprotected. Anyone could hurt him. But who would ever be able to hurt someone so small, so faint, so diminished?

When I whisper good-night my father's jaw moves as if he's chewing. "An involuntary reflex," my husband whispers, not wanting to wake him. All the months, years, since I told my husband what my father did to me, he's hated him, has been capable of anger toward my father that I haven't yet been able to reach. But right now even he, watching my father, seems to find it difficult to sustain it.

As we turn off the lamp, my father's jaw is still chewing.

The next day Mack, Kiki, her daughter Sarah (Todd, my nephew, has not flown up here), and I sit in the lounge making arrangements for the memorial service. Sarah sits beside me on the couch, leaning her head against my shoulder. I slip an arm around her. Still young, in her early twenties, she seems exhausted with the family crisis, maybe scared of this death, scared of her grandfather's dementia. Just scared. She has come to me for reassurance, for comfort. I want to give it. Always I want her to know how much I love her. And for a moment I think about that winter night Todd was born in Boston, and how I felt, for the first time in my life, what I can only call love, an ancient love, a need to protect. I felt the same later when Sarah was born, another small treasure, yes, but as babies and children helpless, too, I noticed, when I baby-sat for Todd and Sarah when they were little.

Sarah, now sitting close beside me for comfort, is relaxed. And I realize: *She is not scared of me.* We talk frequently on the phone. Whenever possible I visit, or she, whenever possible, visits me. *She is not scared of me.* She knows she is safe with me, has always been safe, from the moment she was born. I glance at her to check this reality. She smiles at me. I know, I'm sure, she's not scared of me. And suddenly these six words reveal to me a lifetime of lies—my parents' lies.

But truth, too. I see a startling truth: That just because you are molested as a child does not mean you must grow up to be a molester. You do not have to pass it on. I have not passed it on. For what I truly discovered that moment I first saw Todd—discovering, only in a glimpse, at that moment but am discovering more truly now—is that the definition my father had taught me for love, of how to love a child, is wrong. But more than wrong. Simply, yet profoundly, *his* definition has always been absent in me.

And a deeper truth: My father and my mother each had a choice, could have chosen a different definition of love. They could have realized they didn't know how to love their children healthy, love them well. They could have understood their impulse and sought help. Until they recovered, they could have sent Kiki and me to live with my aunt and uncle. They chose to stay together. They were the parents, the adults, they chose to be. We all are the parents, the adults, we choose to be.

I think of last night, of my father's jaw, chewing. Was he chewing in order to swallow? Swallow his grief? Now as he's dying is he grieving, too late, the death of a daughter? Is he grieving the real death of his wife? His wife, my mother. Who was she to him?

He never left her; she never left him. So I must know they *wanted* to remain married all these years, almost sixty. *Daddy, for me?* Did he stay with her in order to stay with me? Or did he stay with her because she was his wife? She *was* his wife, the one to whom he wrote beautiful anniversary letters. Who was I, then? Certainly I wasn't his daughter; certainly I wasn't his wife. A mistress? A lover? A slut? Yes, my mother always called me that. She received the tribute, the money, the title of wife while she allowed me to perform unspeakable acts with her husband, acts she didn't want to perform herself. *Her* love: I was a present to her husband. *His:* how gratefully he accepted me. They chose to be dangerous parents. It is a choice: to choose to protect children or not. To choose a different kind of love or not. Right now I'm angry she's dead, angry because right now I want to kill her.

By the time I go to bed that night, I know my mother's body has been cremated. What is the chill in the black brick oven where her naked body sleeps? It is the steel pallet she's placed on. It is the whoosh of night roiling down the chimney. As the harsh lick of flames devours her body, it is the inner core of her bones cooling the oven. Each strand of hair is ignited, her head a bristle of fire surrounding her face. Her face will be the last to perish. Her toes and fingers curl in heat, her breasts wither. Through the transparent skin on her neck, her throat glows like the glass chimney of a hurricane lantern. I see inside. I see the gaseous venom of her words spew into her mouth like ash. With the force of the sharp syllable "slut," her jaw cracks open and flame explodes, igniting her tongue and her teeth. They burn to soot. Soot dots the corners of her lips. Her eyes, still, are peaceful: She escaped the rage of my father; she desired his rage for me. And she is peaceful now because this—in this black brick oven—is where she has always lived and where she has always wanted to be. Now, no longer can anyone touch her. She dies before I reach my wrath; she dies before I can remind her I'm her daughter.

The next day we receive the ash and bone of my mother. She is inside an 8 × 6-inch black box, 5 inches high. The box is made of heavy plastic and was constructed in Orlando, Florida. The box is too big for her and when I turn it the ash slides from side to side. I hear her sliding. Feel the weight shifting. Attached to the box is a Certificate of Cremation by the Southern Minnesota Crematory, performed by Ron Hodge. A stranger. She would like this, the way she loved to display her body to doctors. Surely her darkest fantasy was to be placed naked by a stranger inside a black brick oven. By a man. By no one she would ever have to know, by no one who would ever know her.

□ □ □

My father remained married to his wife to be with us all: his three precious little girls. By staying with us, he had all three of us dying for his love and affection. Even though he had none, ever, to give us back.

□ □ □

> Father, I want to ask you: What do you remember? I want to ask you: What do you know? How did you first decide to open the door to enter my bedroom? What was your desultory, internal passage through time and space that brought

you to my body, brought you to my bed? I want to ask if you remember what we did behind all the bedroom walls. Where no one could see. When no one was watching. No one saw the curtains barely shudder as you opened the door. Softly. So no one could hear. Or was no one listening? Because no one would want to hear this, ever. Except I heard. To me, your footsteps echoed as if you walked deserted corridors, always coming toward me. The air around you was fierce and tense. It was as thick as heat and unbreathable, combustible, urgent. Because I heard, I remember. And because I remember terror, Father, I remember you.

Father, what do you remember?

What I remember is that we never spoke. That I never uttered a sigh. I—your silent accomplice to unforgivable crimes. Your secret partner in unspeakable sins.

Did you love me, hate me, or think you merely owned me? My body/your possession. What did my skin say to you? Did my skin shudder like the curtains, or was it still, shocked to silence?

You are the core of a red sun. I stand encased in a sheet of burning glass until the sun shatters it. In silence. The pieces fall. You shattered me. You made me fall.

It happened at night.

Secrets happen at night.

I waited for you to come at night. You still come at night. Except now you come in dreams of blood.

It was only in the morning, every morning, we cleaned up the evidence, Father, all that blood. Every morning you and I were grimly clean. And still silent.

I'm asking you, Father, what do you remember? If you say nothing, I will tell you. If you say nothing, I will remind you that *you,* Father, were the one to hurt someone who was faint, who was diminished, who was small.

Your nightdaughter

□ □ □

Six days later my father dies. There will be no memorial service for him. Neither my sister nor I return to Minnesota. He, too, is cremated. His ashes, like my mother's, are kept by my sister.

My father couldn't live without his wife for even a week. People think they died together because they loved each other so much. They died together because they loved to hate each other so much, because they didn't know how to live without it. They were addicted to hate, addicted to destruction. The destruction of their lives' work, their life together, has been completed.

So I couldn't save my father, after all. Urgently, he tried to discover life inside my body. Urgently, I tried to nourish him. Desperately I failed, for it was death he, alone, swallowed.

The Girl on the Beach: Recovered

Now my parents are dead. They can only hurt me again if I let them. Only I can allow this to happen. Except I won't. I can't. It is time to turn my head and gaze in new directions. It is time to practice speaking the new words I have learned, time to hear all the new voices.

"Maybe it's time to recover her," Randy says.

Her. The little girl on the beach. I think of her alone on the beach, waiting. She waits for me, has always waited for the adult me to feed her, clothe her, love her. She has waited for me because she believed one day I would stop starving our body, waited because she knew one day I would be able to prevent anyone from hurting her ever again.

So, yes, it's time to recover her forever, time to understand I'll never lose her.

"Come with me, please," I say to Randy. "Will you help me?"

"Yes," he says. "Tell me how."

I say we must walk toward her, slowly, where she always waits for me to come for her. He must carry the blanket in which to wrap her.

"Okay," he whispers. "I'm ready."

In the distance I see her small form turned toward us, watching for us. Even from here her body scares me. It's too thin, too bruised, too small. Her hair is tangled, her skin sunburned, streaked with salt and with sand. The beach is littered with skeletons of sea creatures cast from the ocean onto this desolate shore. Here, on this beach with no breeze, it's difficult to breathe the stifling air. The little girl must be cooled, bathed, fed. For a moment I am exhausted by the responsibility.

I stop walking. "Maybe I don't know how to fetch her."

"Tell her you'll always keep her safe," Randy says. "That's all she needs to know."

"But she's not wearing any clothes," I say. "She'll feel shy for you to see her."

"I know," he says. "But I won't see her in the way *he* saw her. I'll see she's a little girl who needs us to help her."

"But what will you really *see* when you see her? Her body?"

"I'll see she needs to be covered."

"That's all?"

He nods. "And that she needs to be protected. But you choose now," he tells me. "I'll wait here or come with you—whatever *you* want. That's what you need to know now. It's your body—hers. No one will ever tell you what to do with it again. You choose. You. What do *you* want?"

I know what he says about himself is true. If he approaches her with me he won't see her the way my father did. He'll see her as a hurt little girl.

Yet I say: "I don't know what I want. I don't know how to decide. I've never decided."

"Then this can be the first time—now."

"I don't know, I don't know. Why don't we stop doing this? This beach doesn't even exist. Maybe I'm not ready to get her."

"Oh, believe me," he says. "You're ready. Would you like to try?"

I glance at her. I glance at Randy. This is about trust, of course. Do I trust him? Do I trust myself?

"Okay," I say. "I want—" I hold out my hand. "Maybe if I carry the blanket. I'll wrap it around her. But I think, yes, I want you please to come with me."

By the time I reach her and wrap her in the blanket, she's sleeping. I carry her back along the beach, but as I grow tired I ask Randy if he'll help me. He takes her from me. Her head nestles against his shoulder, sleeping. A small breeze blows her curls. Her mouth is barely parted, breathing. She must be too warm in the blanket, for she stretches out her arms and wraps them around Randy's neck. Her arms, her elbows, her wrists, her hands, her fingers, snuggle closer. Finally, we are safe.

She and I are alone in a house. We sit in a room of sunlight. Outside is a field of tall grass and a cleansing breeze blows the scent of an azure sky through the open windows. Curtains shimmer. She wears a cotton dress the color of limes. Her feet are bare. She wants to feel the grass under her soles when we are ready to go outside. First I must brush her long hair free of tangles. I brush it until it shines, but carefully, scared I'll hurt her. She is beaming. Her dark lashes blink in the unaccustomed breeze. Surrounding us, in every particle of air, is Randy's presence, as if his copper-colored skin and his blue-blue eyes can bathe us in sweet-scented warmth. He has warmed us. He has given us life.

GREEN

Christmas Spirits

When I enter the classroom I notice her immediately. She is obese and has difficulty fitting onto the school chair attached to the desk. She wears thick glasses, and the skin on her face is pale as if she hides from sun, hides from light. Stringy hair trails to her shoulders. Her clothes, not just because of her weight, are ill-fitting, the material worn and beaded. She looks unsure, awkward, ashamed, defeated. And *this* is why I notice her immediately: because I remember my own awkwardness and shame, as if we are twins. Even though when I starved myself I was skinny, there is no difference between us, for I, too, looked ill-fitted, always expecting to fail.

I put my books on the teacher's desk—*I,* now the teacher, teaching freshman English part-time at a local college. I stand before the class feigning authority, worried that I am *still* ill-fitted, worried that the students will know how I spent my childhood, or will think I'm not a real teacher. Yes, I dress differently now, wearing clothes I hope look professional. Still, I'm scared and unsure.

On this first day I introduce myself, hand out a syllabus, and am more than a little surprised that every student actually *reads* it, only a syllabus, yes, but one I've written. I'm even more surprised that all the students copy down words I write, *my* words, that I write on the blackboard. But maybe it's only because my clothes make me look professional.

When I call roll I learn the name of the obese girl. Kathy. I have this small dread she won't make it.

I've never taught before, and I can't *begin* to figure out prepositions, but I am willfully determined to succeed because I believe I've failed at everything I've previously done. So I'm up at four o'clock every morning to grade papers or prepare classes. By nine o'clock at night, after again grading papers or preparing, I fall asleep, exhausted. I work Saturdays and Sundays, every weekend, grading papers. I read essay after essay, all the essays, very carefully. Because the essays are so personal—more personal than I would have expected—I must, besides correcting grammar, write long notes in the margins and on the backs of pages.

I must respond to my students' tentative, unsure words, words that tell me their stories. They write of alcoholic fathers, of physically violent mothers. Their childhood pets die. Relatives are killed in car wrecks. Best friends die in DUI accidents. As children they are dumped at grandparents' houses as their parents divorce or disappear. One grandmother beats her granddaughter for failing to finish dinner. So I must comment not just about grammar and organization in the margins. I must also express encouragement, or outrage and sympathy. I tell them I'm sorry such terrible things have happened to them. Many don't receive good grades—I grade carefully, fairly—but I must tell them I know, with a little more work, they can do better.

Kathy, whose handwriting is thin and scratchy, writes an essay about all the hours she sleeps. She's scared she'll fall asleep in class and the other students will laugh. As a child, she writes, she always slept in school, at home, in the car, outside on the grass, at friends' houses, before she lost her friends, sleeping anywhere and everywhere. She says she can't stay awake. Her mother used to beat her for sleeping.

And, yes, I understand this sleep. If your body is sleeping, what can it feel? If your mind's not awake, what can it know? I imagine Kathy slumbering through endless summer heat. I imagine white sheets graying after hours and days of sleep. I remember the summer I slept in the West Indies. I remember being engulfed in clouds of sleep. I wonder where Kathy's father is while she sleeps and sleeps and sleeps.

But even when my momma beat me, I couldn't wake up, Kathy writes in her essay. *I could never wake up.*

In the margin of her paper I tell her I'm sad this has happened to her, sad her mother beat her, sad she couldn't wake up.

My students and I don't talk about these things. They write their essays; I respond, by writing and writing in the margins.

I assign the topic of child abuse for one of their essays. I am able to say they can write about physical, emotional, or sexual child abuse, say these words without flinching. "If you need information, you should be able to find magazine articles in the library," I tell my students. I want them, I want everyone, to understand it.

Without explanation, Kathy doesn't turn in the essay. Two days after the deadline I quietly ask her about it. She claims she's hard at work on it and will turn it in Monday.

On Monday, no essay, no Kathy. Now, three weeks before the end of the quarter, this is the first class she's missed. I know, I absolutely know why she missed it.

I check her schedule and meet her after one of her classes. She looks terrified, assuming I'm angry at her for not turning in the essay. I lead her to my office, saying, no, no, you misunderstand, I'm not angry. I close the door and turn on a lamp. "Kathy, please, sit down," I urge her, nodding toward the chair.

She sinks into it and stares down at her scuffed white tennis shoes with split seams. Yes, I stared at my feet during every school confrontation, no matter how mild. Her fingernails are ragged and dirty. Lint flecks her sweatshirt, and behind the thick glasses her eyelids are rimmed with granulated lashes. The skin on her face, as she seems to sway between fear of this encounter and, perhaps, total dissociation, alternates between a dark flush and opaque white, as lifeless as a statue. I want to help her feel better. I want to help her feel at ease. With my linen blazer and freshly ironed blouse, with nylon stockings without runs and polished shoes, with clean fingernails and a showered body, with shampooed hair and jewelry and makeup, how can I ever tell her, *how can I tell you, Kathy, no, no, no, this is not truly me—at least has not always been me. I am not exactly this person you see before you. I have not always been who you think you see.* I want to tell Kathy it might take years of work but she can create a stronger self, too.

But I fear my words will sound false to her. If I'd heard these words from a woman now dressed as I am, I would never have comprehended what that woman was saying.

"You know, when I was in college, I never really felt like other kids." I nod toward the open window where girls sit on new spring grass and pretend to study for finals. As guys pause to talk with them, laughter echoes across the yard. "Even if I hung out with them, I think I was always waiting for someone to tell me to leave."

She looks surprised. Surely this is not what she expected me to say. Slowly she shakes her head. "But you're—" She doesn't know how to finish her sentence. Tears rise slow from the corners of her eyes.

"What is it?" My voice is quiet, almost a whisper. "Can you tell me?"

"It's the essay," she says.

She tells me she hasn't finished it. She tells me she never even started it. Well, she started reading magazine articles but she never began to write it. She lied to me the other day, she says, and she feels so bad. Besides, she still can't write the essay. She'll never be able to write it, even though she knows she'll receive a zero and will probably flunk the course.

"Could you tell me why you can't write it?" I ask her.

I must know the answer before it's given. Her mouth looks as if the skin might crack. "I didn't know—" Her words sound thin, tight. "Till I read this magazine article. On that child abuse. That that's *me*."

The tears are gone. Her words, as she stops speaking, seem gone, as if they landed at the bottom of the sea like tossed rocks. Even in the heft of her body she seems to be draining out of herself, disappearing. "I'm so sorry," I say. "That should never have happened to you."

I'm terrified I've made a terrible mistake by asking Kathy, asking any of the students, to write on this subject, that I'm asking Kathy, in particular, to know something before she's ready. I try to tell her to forget about the essay—it's only an essay. I look in the school directory for the name of the counselor and urge Kathy to make an appointment. This is more important than the essay, I say, nudging a scrap of paper with the counselor's name into her hand. She takes it. Or her fingers manage to hold onto it as I stuff the paper in her fist. I worry that later, when she opens that fist, the paper will slip out unnoticed.

I must do more. I must tell her. As I speak, though, I know she's fading, that maybe she's already gone. I want to urge her back. "Kathy, I want you to know that was me, too, that child abuse. That happened to me, too."

For a moment she seems stunned. Rigidly she seems to nod her head, although I'm not sure she heard what I'd said. She has heaved herself from the chair and is heading toward the door. I go after her into the hall. I point to her fist. I take the paper back and write my own home number on the other side. I tell her to call me. Call me anytime. Day or night. Or call the counselor. Call someone who can help her . . . will she call someone? She nods her head. But she is already gone.

Kathy. I believe one day you will be ready to be helped. And I want to believe you know I have never forgotten you and your secret, that I am with you always while you struggle.

I also must pass you, Kathy. Maybe because I know you will always expect to fail. Maybe because there are times we must receive high marks for simply surviving.

I discover, over the years of teaching, that I most enjoy teaching students who hate English, who hate to write. Most students believe, at least at the beginning of the quarter, they have nothing to say. Our language scares them. Words scare them. Their voices scare them. Grammar terrifies them. Education scares them. Many tell me they're stupid. But when they say this I hear not their voices, but, rather, the imitated voice of an unknowing parent or unprofessional teacher who said this to them first. I tell them they're not stupid. Maybe the parent or teacher didn't know how to teach them, didn't know how to listen, didn't bother enough to care. I urge them to try again. Every quarter I want to see if maybe even one student might change his or her mind, if one student might discover a word, a whisper of a voice, if one student might realize he or she has something that must be said.

Marcia never had anyone to listen to her, never had anyone to care, has always hidden her wishes and her words as if they're secrets. Marcia's face is calm and serene, while her hair is a loose mass of caramel-colored curls, lovely and wild. In class today I'd mentioned I loved words. Now, after waiting for the other students to leave the room, she bends close to me and whispers, "I love words, too." She seems to be holding her breath, her body tense, as if she thinks I'll belittle her admission. I nod, serious, encouraging her. "But I've never told anyone before," she continues. "Everyone I know would've laughed. I mean, I didn't know it was okay to love words."

"But it *is* okay," I say. "I'm glad you love them."

She nods and puts her books on the corner of my desk. "I've kind of been writing poems since I was little, but I've never told anyone or shown them to anyone. I mean, they're not very good."

"I'd like to see them," I say. "If you'd like to show them to me."

She beams and shrugs. "I'm going back to school to be a nurse, but I've always wanted to be an English teacher. I don't mean I could teach college or anything—but maybe middle school. But I don't know. I don't think I'm probably smart enough."

I tell her I think it's great she's found something she loves, that I think she'd be a wonderful English teacher, that she is smart enough. Over the quarter I help her with her writing, with her skills. I give her my phone number and she calls to ask me questions about her life, about her career, about her future. "Am I good enough?" she always wants to know. Yes, I say, you are always good enough, for anything. Finally she switches her major to English. She transfers to a four-year college. She begins to feel confident she can be an English teacher. It never would have occurred to me I could have helped anyone plan a future.

Kathy's story and Marcia's story are only two stories. Over the years there will be more students, other stories. Always, I listen. I must listen. I begin to think that listening and encouraging are more important than teaching punctuation or grammar. Or maybe just teaching students not to fear words, so then they can learn their own words, hear who they are, tell their own stories. At the end of quarters I receive letters and poems, small presents from my students, thanking me . . . mirroring the small offerings and scribbled notes, the tentative words I give Randy, thanking *him,* words that gradually are woven into my story—while Randy's words, in turn, offer me safety, offer me life. So with Randy, with my students, I must thank them, for with them, all of them, I begin to see and hear the circular interconnectings of poems, words, people, scraps of paper, voices, all woven into a strong tapestry to cloak the earth in comfort. Individual threads knit together to form a strong fabric. And I know this can be the way the world is now.

□ □ □

I join a gym to use the weight-lifting equipment. I bench press, execute bicep curls, leg curls, sit-ups. Over the weeks and months I add more and more bars of weight to the stack. I learn the names of my muscles: triceps, quadriceps, deltoids, biceps. I stand before a mirror and notice small curves swelling beneath my skin. I touch my muscles. I flex. I am amazed by these muscles I have created. These muscles seem to be tangible evidence of existence, proving I now live inside my body. This is my body. And now only I decide what it wants—no, what *I* want.

□ □ □

Finally, my sister and I are orphans. We maneuver through our parents' deaths and look at each other: We survived. When my sister received our parents' ashes, she promised one day she'd carry them to Israel for burial. She will be the one to fulfill this final responsibility of a daughter. I cannot. There's nothing more I can do for them. I think my sister knows this, and I'm grateful.

Kiki knows this because I finally revealed to her the secret of our father. Although I first told her shortly before I entered the hospital, it is only now, after our parents' deaths, that I am truly able to hear the gentleness of her response. It has taken me these two years to trust myself enough to trust her, or trust that, together, we will survive the sound of the word "incest," that this word, spoken aloud, can be tolerated and absorbed into our family history. She was very quiet when I told her, as well as patient, asking few questions, wanting perhaps to know as little as possible. Still, she did not rush off the phone or run away. Rather, her voice was small and scared, her silences tangible with worry. She carefully listened to what I said, even as my own voice faltered, struggling to pronounce the words of this new language. And although I didn't ask directly, she claimed our father had never touched her.

Soon after this initial conversation my sister called my husband one evening while I was in the hospital to tell him she was worried about me and hoped I'd be able to recover. She also told my husband she loved him. "What she meant, what she was saying, I think, is that she loves me because I love you, for being with you and caring for you," my husband later relayed to me. "She also told me how much she loves *you*."

How much my sister loves me. At that time I had trouble hearing those words. Or I heard them, but struggled to understand the meaning. Because every year during our childhood, Kiki and I lost more and more words, until we no longer knew how to speak to each other except with the thinnest of phrases, except with the dissonance of emotional lies. Like motes of dust, our words lie carelessly scattered across a vast expanse of childhood. Now we begin, like earnest children, to learn to speak simple words, words of one or two syllables, words such as "sister," "life," "hear," "speak," "soul." Words such as "love." We must begin here, at the beginning, before we can learn to move on.

One evening, several years after our parents' deaths, my sister calls. She says she saw a cute little girl on the street that morning. "She reminded me of you when you were little. You were such a cute kid," she tells me.

As if I am hearing the sound of her voice for the first time and am stunned by its gentleness, I sink onto the chair next to the telephone. "Thank you," I whisper.

Then it is her voice to go small, her voice to sound like a small girl, a sound I don't remember hearing when she was little. "I feel so bad I couldn't have protected you," she says. "You know, from what he did to you."

"Oh, Kiki, no, no. I mean, that's so sweet. But you were just a kid, too. You couldn't have stopped it. *She* was the only one who could've stopped it." And now, now I must tell her, for now is the time, even though I have told her before, I must tell her again, believing this is the first time she will know what I mean. "I have always loved you, too, Kiki."

Kiki. My sister's real name is Carol. When I first began to speak I couldn't pronounce the sound and formed the word "Kiki" instead. While I have always called her Kiki, I have never been able to hold onto Kiki. The two quick syllables of that nickname exploded beyond my reach and there I was, alone, unable to grasp her, unable to see a fading image, unable to hear a vanishing sound.

Now, I whisper the name "Carol." The two long syllables linger in my mouth. The slow-slow sound "Car-ol" slows my sister. Now

I believe, and must trust, that she can pause to hear the heavy weight of my voice say her name, pause long enough to see me, hear what I must say: *Carol, you have always been my sister.*

And now I believe, deep down, that even as a child Carol always loved and missed me, too. But because of our parents, she wasn't able to show it. Now, in the soundlessness of their deaths, in the infinite stillness of their absence, I believe my sister and I will learn to hear each other better.

□ □ □

I volunteer at a shelter for battered women. I am in a house where windows and doors have double and triple locks to prevent angry men from entering. I've never seen any man enter, never seen any man in this house. It is a haven for women and children who need a safe place to heal, a place to hide.

The director of the shelter and I serve dinner to the women and children. We have set the table in the dining room: plates, silverware, napkins, glasses. I'd stopped at Kroger and bought a bouquet of flowers for a centerpiece. Staff, volunteers, guests of the shelter and their children—we all eat together, early, because of the children. A late-afternoon sun angles through slats on venetian blinds. Outside, rush-hour traffic rumbles down the street. But inside we are quiet. The click of silverware. The low murmur of voices. No one outside knows we are here, inside. No plaque or sign marks this ordinary house. The address is not listed in the telephone directory. No angry man will ever find us.

I sit across from Jean. Bruises mar her cheekbone, a scab clots her lip. Valiantly, she wears eye makeup, blush, even lipstick, which is gently smoothed across the scab. With narrowed eyes she secretly glances at the director and at me as we cut our food into small pieces, as we place silverware on our plates while chewing, as we use napkins, then replace them in our laps. With tentative movements Jean seems to imitate us, do what we are doing, as if no one has ever taken the time to teach her how to eat.

I imagine my sister here with me. I imagine my mother. I imagine the three of us all here together, somber but safe. I imagine having lived here forever, the one permanent resident in this impermanent flow of women and children drifting through. Every night I would sleep in a room full of beds, beds crammed together, all the little girls safely tucked into their beds while they sleep.

After dinner I sort through bags of donated clothing. I fold women's clothes into separate stacks of small, medium, large. I separate summer clothes from winter clothes. Shirts, blouses, sweaters from skirts and slacks. I separate children's jeans from dresses. In my family, my mother always dutifully donated outgrown or outdated clothes to charitable organizations. I never considered where my clothes actually went or who might eventually wear them. Now I imagine a pile of my childhood clothes here in this house. A little girl retrieves my favorite lime-green dress and wears it.

I discover a pretty silk blouse with pearl-like buttons. I take it to Jean's room, but she's not there. Her suitcase is by the foot of the bed. I fold the blouse and leave it.

I find Jean in the lounge reading the want ads. She lost her job as cashier at a convenience store because her husband, who'd accused her of cheating on him, smashed the door of the store and beat her. Yesterday she had an interview at a fast-food restaurant, but her shoulders seem exhausted with defeat when she mentions the pay is close to minimum wage. She can't support two children on minimum, so she knows she needs to learn some skills in order to get a better job. If she can't, she's scared she'll go back to her husband, who will beat her. She's more concerned he'll start beating her children. She tells me she doesn't see a future.

I sink down beside her on the couch, also scared about her future. But I tell her how brave she is to be here, to have protected herself as well as her children. I say I'm sure, in not too much time, she can learn some skills, maybe take courses at a technical school in order to get a better job to support her children.

The following week I bring her information about training centers. After dinner she sits beside me on the couch to read the brochures. On the floor by our feet Jean's two children play a board game. Another boy, a preschooler named Joey, wanders into the room sucking his thumb and dragging a ragged blanket for security. Without a word he climbs onto my lap. He hunkers against me in a tight curl and closes his eyes.

I stroke his hair. I trail my fingers down his back. I think of my sister, of rubbing her back, the only time she allowed me close to her, the only time she sat still long enough for me to hear her breathing, hear her heart beating. In a moment Joey is sleeping. I wrap my arms around him and press my cheek against the top of his head. His hair smells of shampoo and of sun. I hug him tighter—as if this one hug can dispel all childhood nightmares. I want it to; I know it can't. I want what I can't have: to know, to be sure, he will always be protected.

But he is safe now. Jean and her children are safe now.

This house is quiet. We all seem to speak quietly here, even the children, for we have all heard too much noise outside. From the other rooms trails the slow murmur of women's voices, brave women who have fled their homes and their husbands for the security of this shelter, for themselves and for their children. I listen to them, a comforting blend of voices, listen until I imagine I hear another voice, a murmur of my mother's voice, finally safe with other women, her voice, a sound I long to hear, longing to hear her say one special word, and I must believe I hear her whisper it. It is to me she calls. I hear her say my name, that one soft syllable. She calls to me, telling me she wished she'd found her way here years earlier to claim even one night of safety for her and her daughters.

I will carry this soft sound of my mother's voice home with me, carry all these women's voices home with me, this, as well as the rustle of paper as Jean plans her future. I carry the sound of Joey's sleeping breath home with me, a steady breath which lulls him until morning. These sounds will lull me until morning.

□ □ □

My husband has always wanted for us to buy a house. I have resisted because I feared responsibility, feared the *idea* of home, the only definition of home I had ever known. Finally, agreeing to seek other definitions, I relent. We are busy decorating and fixing up our new home, even though sometimes I feel like a kid playing house.

It is night. My husband is sleeping. I sit in this quiet house surrounded by my parents' possessions. I sit on their navy and tan couch. Silk material my father bought in the Orient has been sewn into curtains. Their vases, candlesticks, books, lamps, and photograph albums decorate mantels, bookcases, coffee tables. My blankets are in their antique trunks.

But their possessions aren't them. Their possessions are merely lovely things to admire. This is not their home. This is not their house.

It is night, a peaceful Christmas night. The lights on our Christmas tree, the scent of pine, warm the living room. Earlier my husband and I drove to the Christmas tree lot where I lingered, admiring every tree. I wanted to carry all the beautiful trees home with me, place a tree in every room, beside every window. Finally we settled on one, thick and sturdy.

So now *we* are that family to slide our tree into the back of our station wagon. Now my husband and I are that family to hang red, green, silver, gold metallic balls on our tree. We string blinking lights. Strand by strand we drape tinsel from each bough. My husband has a painted tin bird, a Christmas ornament saved from his childhood, that we clip onto the tree. While we want this childhood ornament, a precious heirloom, to connect us to children, to who we were as children, still, we secure the bird to *our* chosen tree, in *our* chosen house, to *our* lives, lives that we now choose to be gentle.

Christmas lights sparkle on the tin bird, reflect on winter windows, sparkling until the bird seems to be ruffling its feathers, fluttering. I imagine it circling the tree, then flying out through the window. I watch it soar over yards in the neighborhood, down the street and across town, far beyond. I imagine the bird winging back to my first Christmas tree that I secreted in my bedroom in New Jersey, back to that night of Christmas spirits that watched over children, protected us from night, this bird revealing to me how far it's possible to fly—from that treasured tree back then, forward, to this tree now.

On this Christmas night I am with my cat Quizzle, who curls on the floor by the tree. Quizzle is still leery of designs in Oriental carpets, but I firmly believe one day she'll trust that the designs don't camouflage coiled serpents, fanged snakes. Besides, Quizzle is much more than her fears. She's in touch with her "inner kitty" and loves to play. I strip edges off computer paper and unfurl them, heaping them into a mound on the floor. Quizzle races across the room and leaps onto them, as if they are autumn leaves. She rustles her way to the bottom and hides. I pretend to search for her. She purrs and purrs when discovered.

Now I stroke her luxurious gray fur, the color of a comforting shadow. I scratch her chin. Her purr comes quick and seems to twine with the warmth of Christmas lights, both trailing down the hall to the rest of the house. I listen. Her purr rises from her throat, rises into the house, rises into this Christmas night, this purr, purr, purring, a soft, steady sound of joy and connection which can be the living center of the house if I let it. And I will. I want to tell Randy. If Randy were here I would whisper, *Randy, this is what you mean, isn't it? This is what you mean. This peace is love; these connections are life.* But I will wait for Tuesday to tell him. Every Tuesday we still learn together, more and more, about this kind of love, this kind of life.

I lift Quizzle and carry her down the hall to the bedroom. Quietly, I open the door. It is dark and warm, but safe.

Mack stirs and lifts his head. "What?" he says. "What's wrong?"

With me, he always expects disaster.

"Nothing," I whisper. "It's me and Quizzle. We're lonely. Nothing's wrong."

He reaches his steady arm out to us, both of us, and pulls us close, pulls us toward him, to keep us secure against night. Here, he will hold us all night.

Softly I whisper his name. Softly I say, "I'm sorry. You know?"

"All that matters," he says, "is that everything's going to be all right. We're going to make it."

Yes, I'm going to make it. We're going to make it. Mack and me and Quizzle.